ANESTHESIOLOGY: TODAY AND TOMORROW

DEVELOPMENTS IN CRITICAL CARE MEDICINE AND ANESTHESIOLOGY

Prakash, O. (ed.): Applied Physiology in Clinical Respiratory Care. 1982.
ISBN 90-247-2662-X.

McGeown, Mary G.: Clinical Management of Electrolyte Disorders. 1983.
ISBN 0-89838-559-8.

Scheck, P.A., Sjöstrand, U.H., and Smith, R.B. (eds.): Perspectives in High
Frequency Ventilation. 1983. ISBN 0-89838-571-7.

Stanley, T.H., and Petty, W.C. (eds.): New Anesthetic Agents, Devices and Monitoring Techniques. 1983. ISBN 0-89838-566-0.

Prakash, O. (ed.): Computing in Anesthesia and Intensive Care. 1983.
ISBN 0-89838-602-0.

Stanley, T.H., and Petty, W.C. (eds.): Anesthesia and the Cardiovascular
System. 1984. ISBN 0-89838-626-8.

Van Kleef, J.W., Burm, A.G.L., and Spierdijk, J. (eds.): Current Concepts in
Regional Anaesthesia. 1984. ISBN 0-89838-644-6.

Prakash, O. (ed.): Critical Care of the Child. 1984. ISBN 0-89838-661-6.

Stanley, T.H., and Petty, W.C. (eds.): Anesthesiology: Today and Tomorrow.
1985. ISBN 0-89838-705-1.

ANESTHESIOLOGY: TODAY AND TOMORROW
Annual Utah Postgraduate Course in Anesthesiology 1985

edited by

THEODORE H. STANLEY, M.D., and W. CLAYTON PETTY, M.D.

Department of Anesthesiology
The University of Utah Medical School
Salt Lake City, Utah 84132
U.S.A.

1985 **MARTINUS NIJHOFF PUBLISHERS**
a member of the KLUWER ACADEMIC PUBLISHERS GROUP
BOSTON / DORDRECHT / LANCASTER

Distributors

for the United States and Canada: Kluwer Academic Publishers, 190 Old Derby Street, Hingham, MA 02043, USA
for the UK and Ireland: Kluwer Academic Publishers, MTP Press Limited, Falcon House, Queen Square, Lancaster LA1 1RN, UK
for all other countries: Kluwer Academic Publishers Group, Distribution Center, P.O. Box 322, 3300 AH Dordrecht, The Netherlands

Library of Congress Catalogue Card Number   84 - 25535

ISBN-13: 978-94-010-8714-8   e-ISBN-13: 978-94-009-5000-9
DOI: 10.1007/978-94-009-5000-9

Contents

Contributing Authors

Abram, S.E., MD, Medical College of Wisconsin, Milwaukee County Medical Complex, Milwaukee, Wisconsin, USA.

Ballinger, C.M., MD, Department of Anesthesiology, University of Colorado Health Sciences Center, Denver, Colorado, USA.

Bird, F.M., MD Ph D, Sc D, Bird Institute of Biomedical Technology, Sandpoint, Idaho, USA.

Cahalan, M.K., MD, University of California, San Francisco School of Medicine, San Francisco, California, USA.

Castro, J. de, University of Brussels, Hôpital Saint Pierre, Department of Anesthesiology, Brussels, Belgium.

Fragen, R.J., MD, Northwestern University Medical School, Chicago, Illinois, USA

Hamilton, W.K., MD, University of California, San Francisco School of Medicine, San Francisco, California, USA.

Hare, B.D., MD, Ph D, Department of Anesthesiology, University of Utah Medical Center, Salt Lake City, Utah, USA.

Ostheimer, G.W., MD, Harvard Medical School, Brigham and Women's Hospital, Boston, Massachusetts, USA.

Rogers, M.C., MD, Department of Anesthesiology and Critical Care Medicine, Johns Hopkins Hospital, Baltimore, Maryland, USA.

Rosow, C.E., MD, Ph D, Harvard Medical School, Massachusetts General Hospital, Boston, Massachusetts, USA.

Saidman, L.J., MD, Department of Anesthesiology, University of California, San Diego School of Medicine, San Diego, California, USA.

Stanley, Th.H., Department of Anesthesiology, University of Utah Medical Center, Salt Lake City, Utah, USA.

Winnie, A.P., MD, Department of Anesthesiology, University of Illinois College of Medicine, Chicago, Illinois, USA.

Zimmerman, G.A., MD, Department of Anesthesiology, University of Utah Medical Center, Salt Lake City, Utah, USA.

Zsigmond, E.K., MD, University of Illinois College of Medicine, Chicago, Illinois, USA.

PROLOGUE.   LOOKING BACK--LOOKING AHEAD

C.M. BALLINGER, M.D.

On this Thirtieth Anniversary of the University of Utah
Postgraduate Course in Anesthesiology, it seems timely to
look back. How and why did this program start? What
nourished the idea? What was practice like then? Who was
responsible for the early beginnings and for bringing the
course to where it is today. And finally, what does the
future hold for such courses?

Actually the first course in the fall of 1955 came as a
result of urgings by the American Society of Anesthesiologists directed at medical school anesthesiology departments.
The Subcommittee on Instruction of General Practitioners,
headed by Dr. Oral B. Crawford, in Springfield, Missouri,
urged us to provide postgraduate education for part-time
physician anesthetists, i.e. general practitioners.

That initial course was a major undertaking for a small
Division of Anesthesiology[*] which then included two full-
time faculty, two Veterans Administration anesthesiologists,
and about 15 clinical faculty, working in private hospitals
in Salt Lake City and Ogden. Without the assurance of a
positive budget balance from previous years and because the
course was actually given one day per week over eight weeks,
we couldn't afford to invite out-of-town speakers. The
local faculty helping with the first course included the
following:

Name   Present Location
Joseph A. Allen, M.D.   Retired, living in Salt Lake City

---

[*](A Division of the Department of Surgery)

Carter M. Ballinger, M.D.	Professor of Anesthesiology, University of Colorado
Hugh O. Brown, M.D.	Deceased
D. Maxwell Butler, M.D.	Deceased
Reynolds F. Cahoon, M.D.	Active Practice in Salt Lake City
Paul A. Clayton, M.D.	Retired, living in Salt Lake City
C. John Christensen, M.D.	Deceased
Leland D. Eggleston, M.D.	Active Practice in Salt Lake City
Mary C. Googe, M.D.	Active Practice, New Jersey
Edward J. Hruska, M.D.	Retired, living in Arizona
Leland O. Learned, M.D.	Deceased
H. Ruth Mershon, M.D.	Active Practice, Oklahoma
Cecil J. Metcalf, M.D.	Deceased
Edward B. Scott, M.D.	Active Practice, California
Eric E. Simonson, M.D.	Retired, living in Salt Lake City
William Stone, M.D.	Retired, living in New Mexico
Jack D. Stringham, M.D.	Active Practice in Salt Lake City

We invited Dr. Scott Smith, the pioneer Utah anesthesiologist, to be a lecturer, but he was busy serving as President of the American Society of Anesthesiologists.

The course was patterned after the New York Postgraduate Assembly, with hospital observation and practice in the mornings and lectures in the afternoons -- when the faculty could get away from their clinical responsibilities. The course was quite basic, trying to provide some basic science background and safe clinical techniques for the brave (?) naive (?) general practitioners providing anesthesia in some of the smaller intermountain hospitals. As a faculty, we had our differences of opinion on the wisdom of teaching better (and more complicated) anesthesia to part-time anesthetists. However, the alternative in some hospitals in those days was anesthesia by laymen such as non-medical non-nurse hospital administrators or even cooks.

Registration for the first course totaled seven prac- titioners. All of the registrants and I could sit around one table for lunch at the old Evans Cafe near the old Salt Lake County Hospital and discuss what they had observed that morning and some of their practice problems. The course registration fee was $50.00. No one was concerned with continuing education credits or making a list of attendees for the IRS.

What was practice like then? We had learned many of the disadvantages of ether and cyclopropane but were still using them. We were beginning to use succinylcholine for relaxation but knew little about its serious side effects. For non-explosive anesthesia we could offer Pentothal, Demerol, N_2O and trichloroethylene, using a non-rebreathing system. Operating rooms were smelly since scavenging had not yet started. If a cardiac arrest occurred, this was treated by squeezing the heart through the diaphragm or opening the chest and directly massaging the heart. Disturbing reports were appearing regarding the safety of spinal anesthesia.

Somehow the second course was scheduled for February (February 13-18, 1956). Even though skiing was not encouraged we soon realized many of the registrants went skiing in the morning instead of observing in hospitals. Our speakers' list was enlarged to include Dr. James Eckenhoff, then Professor of Anesthesiology at the University of Pennsylvania and Dr. Louis Goodman, Professor of Pharmacology at the University of Utah. Dr. Eckenhoff made seven presentations and noted his busy schedule hardly included time for personal hygiene.

By the time of the third course (February 10-13, 1958) our emphasis was beginning to change towards educating practicing anesthesiologists. Our speakers (Dr. Frederick P. Haugen from the University of Oregon and Dr. J. Jay Jacoby from Ohio State University) emphasized safety during anesthesia and regional anesthesia. Our first commercial sponsor, National Cylinder Gas Co., helped lower the course tuition to $40.00. Trying to hold a dinner meeting at the Alpine Rose Lodge was a disaster because of a snowstorm. Some of the audience did arrive in Brighton, but the rest of us gave up and had dinner in the Union Building. Dr. Haugen reminded us he had moved to Oregon to avoid the problems of snowy weather.

The fourth course (February 9-12, 1959) was headed by Dr. Robert Loehning. Lecturers included Dr. William Hamilton from Iowa and Dr. John W. Pender from Palo Alto, California. We had part of the course in Brighton but skiing still was not part of the regular "menu."

The fifth course (February 8-11, 1960) was headed by Dr. Norman Bergman, Chief of Anesthesia at the Fort Douglas VA Hospital. Topics included Recent Advances in Fluothane Anesthesia as well as a demonstration on explosion hazards with cyclopropane, put on by Dr. George Thomas from Pittsburgh, Pennsylvania. More support came from six exhibitors and sponsors -- Astra, Burroughs Wellcome, Deseret, Merck Sharp and Dohme, National Cylinder Gas, and the Foregger Company.

With the sixth course held at the World Motor Hotel (February 6-9, 1961) we encouraged skiing before or after the course and offered optional skiing or hospital observation before the course on two mornings. Visiting speakers included Dr. Joseph Artusio from New York City, Mr. Wayne Hay from Madison, Wisconsin, Dr. M.T. Jenkins from Dallas, Texas and Dr. Henry Price from Philadelphia, Pennsylvania.

Gradually the course grew in size, more full-time anesthesiologists began coming, the emphasis on general practitioners declined, interest in skiing increased, and the direction for the course was placed in the hands of Dr. Richard Elwyn for fourteen years. He tried various arrangements of having the course at the new Medical Center (which was crowded and awkward, away from hotels and skiing), holding it at the Cest Bon Lodge in Park City (where the facilities were crowded and not conducive to lectures), having it at Snowbird (where the road was sometimes closed and the facilities for lectures and exhibitors were limited), and staying downtown at the Hotel Utah Motor Lodge. Finally in 1978 when Dr. Elwyn passed on the course direction to Dr. Stanley and the new conference facilities at the Hotel Utah became available, arrangements for convenient skiing by using busses for quick transportation

to the slopes were worked out. The course had really arrived
to hold a unique position among CME courses in Anesthesiology.

Certainly it is difficult to sufficiently recognize all
those people responsible for making this as successful a
course as it is today. Each successive course chairman -
myself, Dr. Bergman, Dr. Loehning, Dr. Elwyn, Dr. Stanley,
Dr. Petty -- has made a contribution to its success. Mr. Ed
Lauder, who helped with many of the physical and fiscal
arrangements, the many faithful secretaries and staff assistants
(including Mrs. Rachel Melville, Mrs. Mollie Sato, and Mrs.
Vicki Larsen) the exhibitors, speaker and dinner sponsors, and
the Utah State Society of Anesthesiologists also deserve much
credit. But most of all the faithful registrants (some of
whom have attended 20 more courses) deserve much credit for
their support over the years.

What does the future hold? With the advent of personal
computers, video recorders and players, closed circuit tele-
vision, and other technology, perhaps future CME will be
provided so rapidly in the doctor's home or hospital conference
room so that annual conferences will become obsolete. Rising
travel costs, increasing competition, decreasing physician
incomes, and a less generous tax system may price CME (as we
know it today) out of the reach of many anesthesiologists.
Increasing specialization may require attendance of specialized
courses or use of special CME materials and techniques more
readily available in hospitals. Practitioners may want to
get "hands on" experience with special techniques in short
residencies or retraining programs. Lectures are increasingly
becoming obsolete methods of education since the audience
plays such a passive role in the process.

But on balance I am still enthusiastic about this course --
its overall format of lectures by outstanding speakers from
across the world, carefully prepared lecture summaries in a
convenient book, convenient skiing at well run resorts, and
frequent opportunities for interaction with speakers, exhibitors,
and other practicing anesthesiologists. Together they create
a favorable environment for learning and recharging our

6

enthusiasm for carrying out our anesthesiology responsibilities
on our home turf (hospitals).

In conclusion -- Congratulations Dr. Stanley, Dr. Petty,
Dr. Wong, and your many colleagues for continuing a long
tradition of exciting educational courses and best wishes for
your (its) continued success.

Carter M. Ballinger, M.D.
 formerly Chairman of the
 Division of Anesthesiology
 University of Utah and now
 Professor of Anesthesiology
 University of Colorado Health
  Sciences Center
 Denver, Colorado

CHOICE OF AGENT - TODAY AND TOMORROW

WILLIAM K. HAMILTON, M.D.

From the very beginnings of Anesthesia, arguments have occurred
as to the choice of a proper anesthetic agent. As far as is
easily discernable, all arguments have raged without evidence -
at least in an organized form - upon which to base any side of
the dispute. From ether versus chloroform through the current
narcotic versus vapor controversy, only nitrous oxide has survived and it is now threatened by some. The argument against
nitrous oxide continues a pattern of existing without any evidence at this time that available options provide any increase
in safety of outcome.

The widely diverse pharmacology among the menu of available
anesthetic agents and adjuvants invites choice. It seems so
logical to avoid myocardial depressants - who wants a depressed
heart? It seems entirely rational to proscribe drugs which
increase intracranial pressure. It must be true that an agent
which results in DNA depression is unacceptable. This list
can go on and on - but - it is also logical to note that myocardial depressants have been excellent and safe anesthetics
even for sick hearts; that halothane ushered in the most rapid
growth and development of intracranial surgery; that N_2O has
not been observed to be "toxic" in nearly 1½ centuries of extensive clinical use.

Our specialty - with help from others - has detected badness
in many drugs which have been introduced as friendly agents - and
then ushered them from use. These interlopers include chloroform, cyclopropane, trichlorethylene, diethylether, divynil ether,
methoxyflurane, ethylene, etc. Some had specific undesirable
effects on clinical course and many have been discarded because
of fire and explosion hazards. Additionally specific contrain-

dications have been identified such as the succynil choline - K^+
affair. Definite problems were associated with definite drugs
although they often required many, many exposures for identification. This gives reason for confidence in our ability to
detect badness in drugs.

On the other hand, many cyclical changes in fashion have been
observed which demonstrate the fallacy of our proposals that
drug X is indicated or contraindicated in specific situations.

Narcotics were emotionally contraindicated for neurosurgery
in the 1940's and 50's. The vapors were contraindicated - in
favor of narcotics - for the same procedures in the 70's and
early 80's. I note the vapors are now getting some favorable
press from our neuroanesthesia fraternity - perhaps another cycle
is starting. Cyclopropane and ether were alternately blessed and
damned as agents for cardiac patients, asthmatic patients, and
perhaps other disease states. Various vasopressors have had
intermittent ups and downs as favored approaches to a variety
of circulatory abnormalities. Blood pressure maintenance itself
has had inconsistent recommendations based on seemingly logical
grounds. This cyclical repetition of opposing views at least
argues for inaccurate original base for opinions expressed.

The reasons why the apparently sound arguments do not hold
true include:

a) Causes for outcome variation in the entire surgical exper-
    ience are so varied and large that drug variations are
    overridden as detectable causes for change.
b) Drug actions are classified as if they were pure. In fact,
    however, they are varied and in some part unknown.
c) The human organism and disease states are ultra complex
    and defy one to one matching.
d) Combinations of drugs in variable doses are almost always
    used giving rise to an infinite variety of effects.
e) Variation in operator (anesthetist) perception and reaction
    regarding drug effect offers another variable of infinite
    dimension, rendering prediction difficult if not impos-
    sible.
f) Outcome data are more difficult to obtain than the act of

"predicting" what we believe ought to happen.

In view of the above observations, we in Anesthesia do ourselves and our specialty harm in assigning and defending a specific choice of anesthetic agent for specific disease states or conditions. Not only do we support malpractice litigation and cast an image of immaturity, we impede teaching and research by stating with definity that which is in reality only supposition.

METABOLIC FUNCTIONS OF THE LUNG:
BIOCHEMICAL ACTIVITIES THAT HAVE CLINICAL SIGNIFICANCE

Guy A. Zimmerman, M.D.

The respiratory function of the lung has been recognized for at least three centuries. However, the non-respiratory activities have been emphasized only relatively recently. The large surface area of the alveolar capillaries membrane, and the strategic position of this capillary bed in the circulation, affords the lung a unique ability to perform metabolic activities that have systemic as well as local effects. The metabolic activities of the cells of the alveolar-capillary unit may also be important because these cells are situated at the interface between the external environment and the internal milieu.

The major organ-specific functions of the lung are as follows:
1. Gas exchange.
2. Cellular defenses against toxic elements in the atmosphere; interaction with the environment.
3. Synthesis and maintenance of connective tissue matrix of the lung.
4. Synthesis and maintenance of bronchoalveolar lining material.
5. Metabolism and release of locally-active and circulating polypeptides, mediators, and hormones.

The gas exchange and defense functions of the lung are well known. The extent to which biochemical and metabolic activities of lung cells contribute to these functions is, however, often overlooked. In addition, metabolic activity of lung cells may contribute to other processes that have clinical importance. The remainder of this chapter is an overview of some of these activities, together with speculations concerning their clinical relevance.

The extent of the metabolic activity of the whole lung is partially illustrated by the way in which the mixed venous blood is modified en route through it (1-6,10,19-20,36,45). In addition to a change in oxygen tension and saturation, the blood may be modified in a variety of ways:

1. <u>Materials cleared from the blood by the lungs</u>:
   <u>Completely cleared</u>: serotonin, bradykinin, prostaglandins (E & F series), steroids (cortisone, testosterone), glucagon, ATP, ADP, drugs (propranolol, others).
   <u>Incompletely cleared</u>: norepinephrine, histamine, prostaglandin A series.
2. <u>Activated in passage or secreted</u>: angiotensin I, prostacyclin (controversial).
3. <u>Unchanged in passage</u>: epinephrine, angiotensin II, vasopressin, oxytocin, vasoactive intestinal peptide.

Clearance of circulating agents by the lung involves several different mechanisms (i.e. conversion by cell surface membrane-bound enzymes, as with bradykinin, or uptake and degradation, as with prostaglandins of the E & F series). The specificity of the clearance mechanisms indicates an exquisite level of recognition and control (as an example, the uptake and degradation of norepinephrine but not epinephrine). Although the physiologic significance of most of these activities are still in question, many have potential pathophysiologic significance in disease states. An example is the fact that histamine and norepinephrine cause increased transcapillary fluid filtration in the Staub sheep lung lymph fistula model under the appropriate conditions (8). Thus, impaired uptake and degradation by the injured lung may cause local accumulation of these agents, contributing to pulmonary edema (8).

Since the lung parenchyma depends on energy to perform its metabolic activities (3,9,25-26), hypoxia and decreased blood flow may impair or alter clearance functions of the lung. Other perturbations that appear to alter these activities in whole lungs include the composition of the inspired gas, the level of alveolar ventilation, the pattern of ventilation, and factors that contribute to the mechanical deformation of lung tissue.

In addition to processing circulating materials, the lung parenchyma is able to release agents that may serve as <u>local or systemic mediators of inflammation</u>. These mediators include complement fragments, thromboxanes, and leukotrienes (39). There is a great deal of interest in the production of these and other autacoids in diffuse alveolar-capillary injury, anaphylaxis, and other pathologic processes (Zimmerman GA,

"Adult respiratory distress syndrome: mechanisms and management," in this volume).

The cells of the terminal lung units ("alveolar capillary membrane") probably carry out the bulk of the metabolic functions of the lung (6), just as they are the major contributors to the gas exchange and water exchange activities of this organ. The remainder of this discussion will focus on two specific cell types, the pulmonary endothelial cell and the Type II alveolar cell, as examples of metabolizing, active cells that demonstrate some of the general principles of non-respiratory activities discussed above. Each carries out functions that may be clinically important to the anesthesiologist and intensivist.

The Alveolar Type II Cell and Metabolism of Alveolar Lining Material: The alveolar Type II cell is the most numerous and metabolically-active of the alveolar lining cells (11). Its major functions are thought to be synthesis and secretion of components of surfactant, and proliferation and differentiation in response to lung injury. Other potential functions include: 1) antioxidant defenses, 2) secretion of enzymes and other components of the alveolar lining material in addition to surfactant, which may be important in alveolar defense; and 3) control of the electrolyte composition of the alveolar subphase (11,12). The most well-studied of these processes is surfactant production. The pulmonary surface-active material, or "surfactant," is found at the air-liquid interface of the lung and is responsible for lowering the surface tension at this interface (13). If unopposed, such surface tension would promote alveolar collapse at the end of expiration and result in atalectasis and regional inequality of alveolar volumes, both contributing to disordered gas exchange (12,13). Thus surfactant contributes to the ability of the lung to maintain a stable functional residual capacity, a requirement for normal gas exchange. In addition, surfactant influences permicrovascular pressure and therefore transcapillary fluid exchange (18), acts as an alveolar integumentary barrier, facilitates the clearance of inhaled particles, and enhances the bactericidal capacity of alveolar macrophages (13). The consequences of a surfactant deficit are well-known in neonates with the infant respiratory distress syndrome, the only human disease clearly attributable to surfactant lack. Abnormalities of surfactant composition and biophysical function also occur in the adult respiratory distress syndrome (46).

Surfactant is a biochemically-complex material that is rich in phosphatidylcholine, and is unusual because of the high proportion of saturated fatty acids that it contains (2 palmitic acid [16:0] residues) (12). In addition to phosphatidylcholine, other components, including proteins, are essential for its physiologic function. The exact molecular basis for the synthesis and release of surfactant is unknown, but production and organization of the components occurs in the endoplasmic reticulum of the Type II cell and the surfactant is stored in organelles known as lamellar bodies (11-13). These are secreted by exocytosis onto the alveolar surface and the surfactant is arranged as "tubular myelin", a unique physical form that appears as a lattice structure on electron micrographs (14). The tubular myelin then adsorbs to the air-fluid interface and assumes a different physical conformation with the typical linear appearance (11-13). This conformation appears to be required for the normal ability of the material to lower surface tension. Control mechanisms for surfactant release and metabolism are not well understood, but Type II cell activity is affected by certain hormones and by the pattern of ventilation (3, 11-13). There is also evidence that alveolar Type II cells may take up surfactant from the alveolar surface and reprocess it for later secretion.

Recent investigation of the effects of the pattern of ventilation on surfactant activity has suggested extraordinary qualities of the material that may be of clinical import. While studying the mechanism for decreased lung compliance during constant tidal volume ventilation with low or normal tidal breaths, Thet, Massaro and co-workers found that this pattern of breathing resulted in increased amounts of surfactant in the aggregated form, of which tubular myelin is one physical configuration (14, 15). In the aggregated form the chemical composition of surfactant is the same, but the physical state prevents the surfactant from rapidly diminishing surface tension (17). The development of an increased fraction of aggregated surfactant results in increased alveolar surface tension in normal, excised animal lungs (14, 15, 17). These findings suggest that an alteration in the physical and biologic properties of surfactant can be caused by the pattern of ventilation, a concept developed earlier by Clements (13). Such alterations may explain the atalectatic, liver-like lungs that were observed in animals subjected to constant volume ventilation by Drinker and other early investigators of physiologic alterations caused by mechanical ventilation (16). Thet, Massaro et al reported that the amount of aggregated surfactant can be returned to normal by a single deep breath (approximately 3 times normal tidal volume), and its formation appears to be prevented by a) a periodic sigh during that constant normal tidal volume ventilation, b) continuous ventilation at two or three times the normal tidal volume or c) by the addition of positive end expiratory pressure to continuous normal volume ventilation (14, 15, 17).

Considering these observations, it is possible that alteration in surfactant function caused by an abnormal pattern of breathing may explain the propensity for atalectasis in postoperative abdominal and thoracic surgery patients, whose pattern of ventilation is routinely one of low constant tidal volumes without sighs. Since increased surface tension appears to favor alveolar fluid accumulation (18), the amount of aggregated surfactant may also be important in the genesis of pulmonary edema in some circumstances. Alteration in the amount of aggregated surfactant has been proposed as a mechanism for ventilation-perfusion abnormalities in pulmonary embolism, oxygen toxicity, and the adult respiratory distress syndrome (17).

If the studies that indicate improvement in surfactant function by alteration in the ventilatory pattern (discussed above) are substantiated in humans, they may provide a cellular, biochemical and biophysical basis for common respiratory therapy practices in the operating room and intensive care unit. These include the use of larger than normal tidal volumes during mechanical ventilation, use of the sustained maximum inspiration ("incentive spirometry") in postoperative care, and the use of positive end expiratory pressure in some circumstances.

Synthetic and partially-purified natural surfactants have been administered to humans for the treatment of lung disease. The initial evaluation of these studies indicates that this approach may be useful in premature infants at high risk for severe respiratory distress syndrome, encouraging additional clinical investigations (47).

Pulmonary Endothelial Cell Activity: Many of the metabolic functions of the lung, especially those related to clearance or modification of circulating agents, are carried out by the pulmonary endothelial cells (1-6, 19). Thus the rather simple morphology of this cell is deceptive, because it is extremely active in modifying plasma components. Two morphologic features facilitate interaction of this cell with the plasma. Endothelial cells of the larger pulmonary arteries, and to a lesser extent the capillaries, have abundant surface projections (20) that increase their surface area several-fold. Secondly, the plasma membrane is densely concentrated with "caveolae intracellulares" (pinocytotic vesicles), many of which open onto the lumen of the vessel and increase the surface area (2, 19). These two microanatomic structures contribute to an extensive surface for interaction with plasma, just as the alveolar surface presents a large area for gas exchange (6). The pulmonary capillary surface area has been estimated at 70 M^2 but is probably at least twice that because of surface projections and caveolae; the ratio of the capillary surface area to the volume of blood contained in it appears to be extraordinarily large (19). This feature not only facilitates modification of the plasma by endothelial cells, but probably makes the endothelium more susceptible to injury by blood-borne agents.

The potential for biochemical activity by pulmonary endothelial cells is indicated by the substances that they metabolize or synthesize (19): lipids and chylomicrons, components of the coagulation and fibrolytic system (including a plasminogen activator, factor VIII antigen, and thromboplastin-like activity), biogenic amines, nucleotides, prostaglandins and prostacyclin, and kinins and angiotesins. Several of these processes have been suggested to have clinical import, especially in lung injury states. Two will be mentioned in more detail.

Kinin and Angiotensin Metabolism: In 1967 Ferria and Vane reported that bradykinin was virtually completely eliminated in a single pass through the pulmonary vascular bed. Radioactive bradykinin is hydrolyzed at as many as five of its eight peptide bonds during passage through the pulmonary vasculature, and all of the radioactivity is recovered in the pulmonary venous effluent (19). These, and other, features of bradykinin metabolism strongly suggested that it is hydrolyzed by enzymes on, or near, the luminal surface of pulmonary endothelial cells. In other experiments, infusion of radiolabeled angiotensin I resulted in angiotensin II-activity in the pulmonary venous effluent and recovery of all radiolabeled fragments, implying hydrolysis of the parent compound to the more active principle (angiotensin II) at the endothelial surface (2, 6, 19). It is now known that a lung enzyme, angiotensin converting enzyme (ACE, kininase II) hydrolyzes both bradykinin and angiotensin I (2, 19). ACE is a dipeptidyl carbo-xypeptidase that is found on the luminal surface of endothelial cells when specific antibodies are used to identify its cellular location (19). It is not unique to lung endothelium. However, the pulmonary vascular bed appears to be the major site of degradation of bradykinin and conversion of angiotensin I to angiotensin II. Also, the pulmonary vascular bed is the only one yet studied that does not also inactivate angiotensin II, suggesting that the lung contributes a humoral factor to the systemic circulation that is important in the regulation of blood volume and vascular tone (2, 19).

These observations may be revelant to conditions encountered in the operating room and intensive care unit. Although not proven, altera-tions in ACE activity have been suggested to be important in the im-paired reflex vasoconstriction demonstrated by hypoxic humans, and the inability to increase systemic vascular resistance in response to shock in some individuals with emphysema. This speculation is supported by the observation that degradation of bradykinin (a potent hypotensive agent), and conversion of angiotensin I to angiotensin II (a potent vasocontrictor), are both greatly decreased by ventilation of experi-mental animals with hypoxic gas mixtures. Depression of ACE activity in isolated endothelial cells in tissue culture occurs when the cells are subjected to hypoxic conditions (26), providing an explanation for these findings. Recent studies also suggest that abrupt reoxygenation of animal subjects that were previously hypoxemic and hypovolemic (as in hemorrhagic shock) may cause a "rebound" increase in angiotensin II levels, resulting in impaired coronary and splanchnic blood flow (48). This observation suggests an explanation for the impaired cardiac and bowel function that may be seen as sequelae of shock.

Angiotensin converting enzyme activity has also been evaluated as a marker for endothelial cell injury after cardiopulmonary bypass, and in diffuse alveolar capillary lung injury (ARDS) (27-29).

Prostacyclin Production: Isolated, perfused lungs have the capacity to metabolize arachidonic acid to yield precursors of prostaglandins, thromboxanes and other products (19). Animal pulmonary endothelial cells in culture metabolize labeled arachidonate to at least four products, including two with chromatographic features suggestive of 6-keto-PGF$_1$ alpha and thromboxane B$_2$, which are degradation products of prostacyclin (PGI$_2$) and thromboxane A$_2$, respectively (19). Human pulmonary endothelial cells in culture have been shown to release PGI$_2$ activity into the medium (30). This is not surprising, since the major product of arachidonate metabolism in macrovascular endothelial cells appears to be PGI$_2$. Prostacyclin synthetase activity is most highly concentrated in the intimal cells of vessels, and decreases toward the adventitia (31). The local production of PGI$_2$ is thought to be one feature that renders the vascular surface non-thrombotic, by virtue of its potent inhibition of platelet aggregation and adherence (32), although it is unlikely that PGI$_2$ release plays a major role in normal, uninjured vessels (42, 49; also see below).

Earlier it was suggested that prostacyclin is a "hormone" that circulates in systemic blood (36), in contrast to other prostaglandins that are efficiently taken up and degraded by the lungs (33-36). PGI$_2$ is not a substrate for the uptake mechanism responsible for removal of other prostaglandins from the plasma by lung endothelial cells (31). Based on bioassay techniques, it was reported that the lung constantly releases small amounts of PGI$_2$ into the systemic circulation, where it achieved a higher concentration than in the venous blood (37, 39). The cellular source of the PGI$_2$ activity in these studies was not identified, but was presumed to be the pulmonary endothelial cell. Increased release of PGI$_2$ activity occurred with hyperventilation, suggesting that the pattern of ventilation may alter arachidonate metabolism by the endothelium (37). The release of PGI$_2$ by the lungs was proposed to be an important systemic control mechanism for platelet-vascular interactions which could be impaired by disease (31, 32, 36). As an example, altered release of PGI$_2$ from the lungs of smokers was suggested to contribute to the propensity for atherosclerotic vascular disease in these patients. More recent studies indicate that PGI$_2$ is not released in the absence of appropriate stimulation of the endothelial cells, and is probably not a circulating hormone (42). However, it may be released in vascular injury states (42, 49). Local imbalances between PGI$_2$ production and thromboxane A$_2$ release (a potent proaggregatory substance for platelets and the most potent vasoconstrictor yet identified) may result in platelet and/or leukocyte sequestration in the lungs of patients with diffuse alveolar capillary injury (39) and may contribute to the vasomotor changes (40) occurring during pulmonary insults such as endotoxemia (41).

Significant increases in systemic arterial PGI_2 concentrations occur after the application of mechanical ventilation in patients undergoing thoracotomy, and during perfusion of the lungs after cardiopulmonary bypass in some patients (50). The data suggest that the pulmonary endothelium releases PGI_2 in response to the mechanical stimulation resulting from positive pressure ventilation and that systemic release of PGI_2 may cause some of the immediate cardiovascular sequelae of mechanical ventilation.

Role of the Endothelial Cell in Regulating Pulmonary Vascular Tone. The pulmonary endothelial cell is required for vasodilation in response to acetylcholine and bradykinin in dogs (44). Although the pulmonary response to certain pharmacologic vasodilators may depend in part on PGI_2 synthesis (43), the responses to acetylcholine and bradykinin are not mediated by cyclooxygenate metabolites of arachidonate (44). The pulmonary vasodilatory response produced by these agents appears to depend on the synthesis of an "endothelium-derived relaxing factor" that is not yet chemically-defined (51). The identification of this factor is likely to significantly change concepts of pulmonary vascular pharmacology. Also, it is possible that the lack of response to vasodilators in some patients with pulmonary hypertension associated with the adult respiratory distress syndrome (and other disorders, such as primary pulmonary hypertension) is a manifestation of diffuse endothelial cell injury and the inability of the damaged endothelial cells to release relaxation factors for smooth muscle.

20

REFERENCES

1. Fishman AD, Peters GG: Handling of bioactive materials by the lung. Parts I and II. N Engl J Med 291:844-89, 953-959, 1974.
2. Heinemann HO, Ryan JW, Ryan US: Is the lung a para-endocrine organ? Am J Med 63:595, 1977.
3. Naimark A: Non-ventilatory functions of the lung. Am Rev Resp Dis 115:93, 1977 (suppl).
4. Junod AF: Metabolism of vasoactive agents in lung. Am Rev Resp Dis 115:51, 1977 (suppl).
5. Said SI: Pulmonary metabolism of prostaglandins and vasoactive peptides. Annu Rev Physiol 44:257, 1982.
6. Ryan US: Structural basis for metabolic activity. Annu Rev Physiol 44:221, 1982.
7. Blitt CD, et al: Pulmonary biotransformation of methoxyflurane: An in vitro study in the rabbit. Anesthesiology 51:528, 1979.
8. Minnear FL, et al: Effects of epinephrine and norepinephrine infusion on lung fluid balance in sheep. J Appl Pysiol Respir Environ Exp Physiol 50:1351, 1981.
9. Fisher AB, et al: Energy utilization by the lung. Am J Med 57:437, 1974.
10. Addonizio VP, Harken AW: The surgical implications of non-respiratory lung function. J Surg Res 28:86, 1980.
11. Mason RJ, Williams MC: Type II alveolar cell. Defender of the alveolus. Am Rev Resp Dis 115:81, 1977 (suppl).
12. Mason RJ, et al: Alveolar type II cells. Fed Proc 36:2697, 1977.
13. Clements T: Functions of the alveolar lining. Am Rev Resp Dis 115:67, 1977 (suppl).
14. Thet LA, et al: Changes in sedimentation of surfactant in ventilated exicsed rat lungs. Physical alterations in surfactant associated with development and reversal of atalectasis. J Clin Invest 64:600, 1979.
15. Thet LA, et al: On the mechanism of alveolar collapse during constant tidal volume (CTV) ventilation. Clin Res 27:494, 1979.
16. Drinker CK, Hardenbergh E: The effects of the supine position upon ventilation of the lungs of dogs. Surgery 24:113, 1948.
17. Massaro D, et al: A hypothesis relating breathing pattern to some forms of the "adult respiratory distress syndrome". Am J Med 69:113, 1980.
18. Albert RK, et al: Increased surface tension favors pulmonary edema formation in anesthetized dogs' lungs. J Clin Invest 63:1015, 1979.
19. Ryan JW, Ryan US: Pulmonary endothelial cells. Fed Proc 36:2683, 1977.
20. Ryan JW: Processing of endosenous polypeptides by the lung. Annu Rev Physiol 44:241, 1982.
21. Heistad DD, et al: Reflex cardiovascular responses after 36 hours of hypoxia. Am J Physiol 220:1673, 1971.
22. Heistad DD, et al: Impaired reflex vasoconstriction in chronically hypoxemic patients. J Clin Invest 51:331, 1972.
23. Cohn JN, Luria MH: Studies in clinical shock and hypotension IV. Variations in reflex vasocontriction and cardiac stimulation. Circulation 34:823, 1966.
24. Stalcup SA, et al: Impaired angiotensin conversion and bradykinin clearance in experimental canine pulmonary emphysema. J Clin Invest 67:201, 1981.

25. Stalcup SA, et al: Inhibition of converting enzyme activity by acute hypoxia in dogs. J Appl Physiol Respir Environ Exer Physiol 46:227, 1979.
26. Stalcup, SA et al: Inhibition of angiotensin converting enzyme activity in cultured endothelial cells by hypoxia. J Clin Invest 63: 966, 1979.
27. Claremont JD, Brantwaite MA: Metabolic indices of pulmonary damage: Changes in angiotensin converting enzyme and alpha$_1$ anti-trypsin activity after cardiopulmonary bypass. Anaesthesia 35:863, 1980.
28. Bedrossian CWM, et al: Decreased angiotensin-converting enzyme in the adult respiratory distress syndrome. Am J Clin Path 70:244, 1978.
29. Casey L: Decreased serum angiotensin converting enzyme in adult respiratory distress syndrome associated with sepsis: A preliminary report. Crit Care Med 9:651, 1981.
30. Johnson AR: Human pulmonary endothelial cells in culture. Activities of cells from arteries and cells from veins. J Clin Invest 65:841, 1980.
31. Monacada S, Vane JR: Pharmacology and endogenous roles of prostaglandin endoperoxides, thromboxane A$_2$, and prostacyclin. Pharmacol Rev 30:293, 1979.
32. Monacada S, Vane JR: Arachidonic acid metabolites and the interaction between platelets and blood vessel walls. N Engl J Med 300: 1142, 1979.
33. Hyman AL, et al: Prostaglandins and the lung. AM Rev Resp Dis 117: 111, 1978.
34. Mathé AM, et al: Aspects of prostaglandin function in the lung. Parts I and II. N Engl J Med 296:850-855, 910-914, 1977.
35. Weir EK, Grover RF: The role of endogenous prostaglandins in the pulmonary circulation. Anesthesiology 48:201, 1978.
36. Gryglewski RJ: Is the lung an endocrine organ that secretes prostacyclin? In Vane JR and Bergstrom S (editors). Prostacyclin, Raven Press, New York, 1979, pp 275-288.
37. Gryglewski RJ, et al: Generation of prostacyclin by lungs in vivo and its release into the arterial circulation. Nature 273:765, 1978.
38. Monacada S, et al: Prostacyclin is a circulating hormone. Nature 273:767, 1978.
39. Fantone JC, et al: Chemotactic medications in neutrophil-dependent lung injury. Annu Rev Physiol 44:283, 1982.
40. Voelkel NF, et al: Release of vasodilator prostaglandin, PGI$_2$, from isolated rat lung during vasoconstriction. Circ Res 48:207, 1981.
41. Hales CA, et al: Role of thromboxane and prostacyclin in pulmonary vasomotor changes after endotoxin in dogs. J Clin Invest 68:497, 1981.
42. Majerus PW: Arachidonate metabolism in vascular disorders. J Clin Invest 72:1521, 1983.
43. Rubin LF, Lazar JJ: Influence of prostaglandin systhesis inhibitors on pulmonary vasodilatory effects of hydralazine in dogs with hypoxic pulmonary vasoconstriction. J Clin Invest 67:193, 1981.
44. Chand N, Altura BM: Acetylcholine and bradykinin relax intrapulmonary arteries by acting on endothelial cells: Role in lung vacular diseases. Science 213:1376, 1982.
45. Geddes DM, et al: First pass uptake of ^{14}C-propranolol by the lung. Thorax 34:810, 1979.
46. Hallman M, et al: Evidence of lung surfactant abnormality in respiratory failure. J Clin Invest 70:673, 1982.

47. Taeusch HW, et al: Exogenous surfactant for human lung disease.
    Am Rev Resp Dis 128:791, 1983.
48. Davidson D, Stalcup SA: Systemic circulatory adjustments to acute
    hypoxia and reoxygenation in unanesthetized sheep.   Role of renin,
    angiotensin II, and catecholamine interactions.   J Clin Invest 73:
    317, 1984.
49. Fitzgerald GA, et al: Increased prostacyclin biosynthesis in patients
    with severe atherosclerosis and platelet activation.   N Eng J Med
    310:1065, 1984.'
50. Edlund A, et al: Pulmonary formation of prostacyclin in man.
    Prostaglandins 22:323, 1981.
51. Furchgott RF: Role of endothelium in responses of vascular smooth
    muscle.   Circ Res 53:557, 1983.
52. Gillis CN, Pitt BR: The fate of circulating amines within the pul-
    monary circulation.   Annu Rev Physiol 44:269, 1982.

NEUROLEPTANALGESIA : YESTERDAY,TODAY,TOMORROW

J.DE CASTRO

1 . INTRODUCTION

Stress and pain produced during surgery give a tremendous rise of nociceptive stimuli input to the CNS. It is the role of anesthesia to protect the brain against these excessive stimuli. The most specific drugs against stress and pain are neuroleptics and narcotics.This is the reason why an anesthesia technique producing neurolepsis and analgesia by the combined use of a neuroleptic and a strong narcotic, has been proposed under the name of neurolept-analgesia (NLA) or neuroleptanalgesic-anesthesia (NLAA) if an hypnotic or N20 is added to the NLA association (1)

2 . NLA YESTERDAY

2.1. The 1959-1962 period

Our investigations to find a new IV anesthesia technique,were started at the University of Brussels in 1957.The most used anesthesia techniques and their importance at that time are listed in table 1.

The lytic cocktail anesthesia or neuroplegia, developed by the french school of Laborit after 1950 (2) was an attempt to use separated compounds for sleep, pain, muscle relaxation and autonomic nervous system paralysis. This technique appears very interesting.

Table 1. Anesthesia techniques used at the Brussels Universitary
         hospital in 1957.

Anesthesia techniques	%
- Inhalation anesthesia (ether)	15
- IV anesthesia :	
thiopentone, curare, N20 (classic)	65
lytic cocktail anesthesia (Laborit)	10
- Locoregional anesthesia :	
local	5
peripheral blocks	3
epidural	1
intrathecal	1

Meanwhile, during the same period, Doctor Paul Janssen's
belgian laboratories had just synthetised new potent narcotics
and new neuroleptics which permitted us to develop a more simple
technique putting the emphasis on deeper analgesia(3).

NLA was first introduced in Lyon, in 1959, at the Congress of
the French Society of anesthesiology by Mundeleer and myself
The new selective IV anesthesia technique, was clearly different
from the classical IV anesthesia and from the lytic cocktail
anesthesia. Indeed, thanks to the use of relative high and potent
opiate doses, a more simple drug association became possible (4).

2.1.1. Drugs . For the initial NLA technique haloperidol, a
neuroleptic of the butyrophenone series and phenoperidine, a pure
potent narcotic derived from pethidine, were used without
hypnotics or inhalation agents.

These drugs were rapidly replaced (1960) by fentanyl and
droperidol, two compounds of a similar group, but with shorter
duration of action (5).

It became possible for patients to undergo major surgery
under NLA without the need for any other drug, initially NLA
indicated that patients had not lost consciousness, but gradually

this terminology has been used almost indiscriminately with NLAA
and the subtle difference between the two states disappeared.

For the USA Thalamonal, a standard formulation of droperidol
and fentanyl, was marketed in 1961. This fixed drug combination
of a long acting with a relatively short acting substance was
rather a handicap than progress. However, it was considered by
the FDA as a prophylactic measure against possible drug abuse of
the narcotic outside the anesthesiological field (6).

Table 2 . Advantages of NLA.

1	- Histamine release	very low
2	- Depression of cardiac contractility	minimal
3	- Cardiac sensitization to catecholamines	no
4	- Autoregulation in brain, heart,kidneys	preserved
5	- Cerebral blood-flow and metabolism	preserved
6	- Tolerance of the endotracheal tube	good
7	- Mechanical ventilation	easy
8	- Renal and hepatic toxicity	no
9	- Awakening at any moment	possible
10	- Antagonists of the narcotic	available
11	- Environemental pollution	no
12	- Trigger of malignant hyperthermia	no
13	- Post-operative analgesia	prolonged
14	- Technique simple,safe,potent	yes
15	- Contra-indications (age,risk,duration)	no

Table 3 . Disadvantages and limitations of NLA.

1	- Thoracic rigidity (without muscle relaxant)	possible
2	- Sympathetic stress reactions,hypertension, tachycardia	possible
3	- Endocrine stress reactions	possible
4	- Post-operative respiratory depression	prolonged
5	- refentanylisation after awakening	may occur
6	- Awareness,recall	possible
7	- Abuse potential	possible
8	- Tachyphylaxis	possible
9	- Anormal resistance,ceiling effects	may occur
10	- Paradoxical neuroleptic effects (anxiety)	may occur
11	- Extrapyramidal symptoms (acathisia,dystonia,tremor)	may occur
12	- Convulsions (after very high narcotic doses)	may occur
13	- Prolonged neuroleptic behaviour	may occur

In our country and in continental Europe the NLA and the NLAA have rapidly assumed an important place in anesthesia (7,8,9,10).

2.1.2. <u>Advantages and disadvantages</u>. These have been reviewed on many occasions (11,12). They are noted in tables 2-3.

Some disadvantages can be avoided without great difficulty (Tab.4), but others are inherent to the pharmacological proper- ties of fentanyl and/or droperidol (13).

Table 4 . Methods for reduction of some NLA disadvantages.

Disadvantages	Can reduced by:
- Thoracic rigidity - Awareness and recall - Prolonged respir. depression and refentanylisation	Continuous muscle relaxation N20 and/or benzodiazepine Mechanical ventilation, Prolonged monitoring,titrated naloxone if necessary.

2.2. <u>The 1962-1982 period</u>

The concept of NLA and NLAA has created interest and the number of publications, congresses and books dedicated to the subject all over the world for more than 25 years are too extensive to be reviewed here (14,15,16).

We rather wish to concentrate our lecture only on personal contributions to the topic. During the past 25 years our anesthe- siological practice has been concentrated finding better and more universal solutions rather than the initial NLA. All the different possibilities in the direction of analgesia and neurolepsis have been explored.

It was soon realised that progress could be made in compounds with still higher specificity and potency and shorter duration of action (tab.5). It was easily shown that high doses of narcotics have real advantages during anesthesia, however these advantages are limited by increasing problems during the recovery period, the use of an antidote also creating new problems.

2.2.1.   Drugs for analgesia.   Pure agonists narcotics.
In dogs under mechanical ventilation, a comparative study of cardiovascular, neurological and metabolic side effects of eight narcotics (pethidine, piritramide, morphine, phenoperidine, fentanyl, alfentanil, sufentanil and lofentanil) has shown that great differences arise according to the drugs and doses used (17).The differences are most evident for high and massive IV doses (tab.5).

Table 5.The potency,toxicity and safety margin of 8 narcotics
in curarized and mechanically ventilated dogs.(17)

	Relative analgesic potency to M *	MED50X20 mg/kg IV	Severe sympathic hyperactivity mg/kg IV	Epileptiform EEG changes mg/kg IV
Pethidine	1/3	9.0	+	20
Piritramide	2/3	4.5	+	30
Morphine	1	3.0	60	180
Phenoperidine	10	0.3	6	4
Alfentanil	30	0.1	1.2	5
Fentanyl	125	0.025	2-10	4
Sufentanil	625	0.005	1- 2	4
Lofentanil	6250	0.0005	1- 5	10

+ = lethal ,   M * = morphine,

Table.5 (2nd part) . Metabolic toxicity and safety margin of 8 narcotic in curarized and mechanical ventilated dogs (17).

	Severe metabolic acidosis mg/kg IV	Safety margin MED50/lowest dose producing side effects
Pethidine	8	0
Piritramide	15	3.3
Morphine	40	13.0
Phenoperidine	4	13.0
Alfentanil	1.25	12.5
Fentanyl	1.25	50
Sufentanil	4	200
Lofentanil	2	2000

The safety margin between toxic effects and doses necessary
for deep surgical anesthesia is directly related to the
analgesic potency.

In man, analogue results have been observed (tab.6).

Table 6.Estimated clinical safety margin of 8 narcotics (17)

Drugs	MED mg/70kg IV	Max. dose mg/70kg IV *	Safety margin
Pethidine	100	300	3
Piritramide	50	400	4
Morphine	10	300	30
Phenoperidine	1	>50	>50
Alfentanil	0.3	>30	>100
Fentanyl	0.1	>10	>100
Sufentanil	0.01	>2	>200
Lofentanil	0.001	?	?

(Patients under mechanical ventilation and full muscle
relaxation).* Maximal dose without severe side effects.

For pethidine and piritramide (two relatively weak analgesics)
it is not possible in ventilated patients to give more than 2-3
times the normal dose without severe side effects.

With morphine and phenoperidine doses of a much higher
equivalent potency may be administered, nevertheless side effects
occur between 3-4 mg/kg IV morphine.

For alfentanil and fentanyl respectively, doses up to 450 and
150 ug/kg can be given.

For sufentanil (the most potent narcotic currently used
in clinical practice) we have administered up to 30 ug/kg without
per-operative problems.

Histamine release, hypotension and increased fluid requirements
are problems encountered with high doses of narcotics with the same
or lower analgesic potency as morphine. The same problems are rare
with the more potent pure opiates and non existant with sufentanil.

We have seen that one of the problems with narcotics in anesthesia is that even very high doses are not always able to avoid awareness and cardiovascular hyperactivity (18,19,20,21).

Agonist-antagonist narcotics.

If a agonist-antagonist narcotic is used for NLA the problem of ceiling effects and safety margin already appears with relatively low doses, for buprenorphine the most potent agonist-antagonist, 2 or 3 X the current analgesic dose is the maximum dose that can be used for anesthesia. Higher doses reverse the analgesic effect and produce autonomic nervous system hyperactivity or convulsions. The agonist-antagonists may be used only for balanced anesthesia or NLA with a low narcotic component and addition of other central nervous depressors (22).

In our opinion, sufentanil is the best choice for major surgery. The shorter duration of alfentanil is an advantage for short interventions, however for routine NLA, the advantages of potency for sufentanil and the short duration of action for alfentanil, appear most clearly if high and/or single doses are used without other drugs. They are less evident in situations requiring repeated doses and drug associations (23). Particular advantages of sufentanil and alfentanil will be discussed in our second lecture.

2.2.2. Drugs for neurolepsis : potentiator-correctors of the narcotics. Some disadvantages of the NLA are due to droperidol. Indeed, efficient stress protection requires relatively high doses of the neuroleptic and such high doses may produce an extrapyramidal syndrome, paradoxical anxiety or neuroleptic behaviour of long duration.

Soon it became evident that neurolepsis can be obtained not only with specific neuroleptic compounds, but also with many other inhibitors of CNS.

The most important drugs investigated by us in association with a potent opiate for NLA are listed in table 7 (24,25,26,27).

Table 7. Drugs used in association with an opiate for NLA.

- Neuroleptic:	Haloperidol,droperidol,haloanisone, Chlorprotixen,prothipendyl.
- Benzodiazepines:	Diazepam,flunitrazepam,midazolam.
- Ganglioplegics:	Thiamine (high doses).
- Alpha-beta adrenergic blockers:	Labetalol.
- Antihypertensive:	Clonidine.
- Calcium entry blockers:	ATP.

Synaptanalgesia . High doses of vit.B1 (100 mg/kg) have weak sedative, and weak analgesic properties and also produce muscle relaxation and potent ganglioplegic effects. If they are associated with a potent narcotic, NLA can be obtained without major problems. Nevertheless, the amounts of thiamine required have been a limiting factor on further development (28,29).

Ataranalgesia . The sedative hypnotic, anxiolytic, amnesic, and stress protecting properties (however, relatively weak compared with neuroleptics) of the benzodiazepines (BZD) allow an efficient enhancement of the narcotic effects. Further the cardiovascular depression is minimal and some drawbacks of the opiates are partially corrected a.o. per-operative thoracic rigidity, awareness and recall. On the other hand, BZD are long acting compounds and post-operative sedation or muscle hypotonia may be long lasting. BZD have not the antiemetic properties of droperidol and they increase the risk of"refentanylisation" (30).

Among the BZD, we prefer midazolam for its water solubility, good stress protection and somewhat shorter activity than diazepam and flunitrazepam.

A dose of 0.3 mg/kg of midazolam allows a substantial decrease in the required fentanyl or alfentanil doses (up to 50%) and produces a satisfactory NLA association (31).

Adrenolytic analgesia . Labetalol, administered in doses of 1-2 mg/kg has useful properties for NLA. The alpha and beta blocking effects reduce the cardiovascular hyperactivity (hypertension, tachycardia) in resistent patients. It produces a reduction of the narcotic dose, an important decrease of the capillary oozing, a good stress protection and a favourable pressure rate product. Changes in cardiac contractility are minimal, MVO2 demand is reduced, exessive bradycardia is not seen. Compared with other adrenergic blockers, the bronchial and arterial constriction tendency of labetalol is weak, so that this drug is not contraindicated in arteritic and asthmatic patients. Central or ganglioplegic properties are nonexistant.

The only problem seen if labetalol is associated with fentanyl or alfentanil, is a need for long post-operative monitoring. The alphalytic effect of labetalol is a long lasting one, however this property is not easily detected by clinical observation. Early warning symptoms of bleeding during the postoperative period may be absent. Hypotension and hypovolemic shock related to this type of NLA have been observed several hours after the end of the surgical intervention (32).

Clonidine. It is a potent inhibitor of the central sympathetic activity. If the drug is associated, in doses of 1-2 ug/kg, with alfentanil or fentanyl, reduced peripheral sympathetic outflow and

32

increase in the vagal tone is noted. Sedation and peripheral
vasodilation is manifest, capillary oozing is reduced. Reflex
hypertension is not seen, but bradycardia may be so great that
atropine becomes mandatory. The duration of the clonidine
action is also long (23).

ATP. After limited attempts with an ATP-fentanyl association,
we have also abandoned this NLA association because excessive
bradycardia and even transient asystolia may appear (33).

Finally, it must be noted that several common drawbacks
are typical for most of the narcotic potentiators (tab.8).

Table 8. Common disadvantages of many potentiators used with a
potent narcotic for anesthesia.

- Specificity	poor
- Controlability	poor
. individual sensibility	high
. duration of action	long
. drug interactions	multiple
- Side effects,occasionally inacceptable	
. disequilibrium of sympathetic NS	may occur
. psychic disorders	id
. muscle hypotonia	id
. reflex stimulation	id
. rebound activity (late)	id

2.2.3. Analgesia/neurolepsis ratio. The dose range of the
neurolepsis compounds is rather low because of the already
mentioned side effects, and because these effects are long
lasting. On the other hand, the dose margin of the potent
narcotics is high and the peroperative advantages of the use
of high doses of opiates are beyond doubt.

Acquiring growing experience with narcotics, we proposed
with Viars in 1968 a pure analgesic anesthesia technique with
loading doses of 50 μg/kg IV of fentanyl, without the use of
hypnotics or neuroleptics (34).

The idea of using a narcotic as a complete analgesic was not entirely new. Bailey, already in 1958 (35), used high doses of morphine for cardiac surgery. Many other US anesthesists , a.o. Lowenstein and Stanley, followed the same direction (36,37, 38,39,40,41,42,43,44,45,46). Soon high doses of morphine gave way to high doses of fentanyl (47,48,49,50,51,52,53,54,55,56,57,58).

The per-operative advantages of pure analgesic anesthesia with fentanyl or alfentanil are high : rapid stress free induction, high stress protection, good tolerance and cardiovascular stability. Myocardial contractility remains unimpaired, even in old and poor risk patients with poor ventricular function undergoing major surgery. However, after our early enthusiasm, some inadequacies of the technique became apparent. Cardio-vascular and sympathetic hyperactivity still occured, mostly in young and fit patients. Unconsciousness was not a constant factor and the post-operative respiratory depression problems were still present.

In patients with coronary artery disease, hypertension and tachycardia increase the myocardial work and the 02 demand in the face of a relatively fixed 02 supply (59). Amnesia and "stress free anesthesia" is not always guaranted by pure fentanyl anesthesia, even if used in the highest doses. Association of a potentiator-corrector to the narcotic remains in the daily practice imperative. For each patient and for each intervention, there is an optimal analgesia/neurolepsis ratio. Unfortunately, this optimal ratio is not always easy to foresee.

2.2.4. Antidotes. Narcotic agonist-antagonists can be used for reversal of narcotic overdose at the end of the surgical

intervention. The pure antagonist naloxone has replaced the
agonist-antagonists. However, benefits of the procedure, even if
naloxone is used in small and titrated doses, cannot outweigh
the drawbacks; it must be reserved for emergencies.

2.2.5. Stress protection. In the early period NLA certainly
went beyond the goal of light and easily reversible anesthesia,
reducing prejudice to stress protection. Complete stress
protection, however, is never reached and is probably not
necessary. Also here, the optimal situation lies between two
extreme solutions, but the right depth for NLA sometimes remains
uncertain.

3 . NLA TODAY

The present NLA technique, just as before, is based on the use
of a potent opiate associated with a potentiator-corrector and
a muscle relaxant. Within this frame, many formulae are at our
disposal.

3.1. Narcotic/potentiator ratio

Modern NLA is performed either with small, medium or high
doses of narcotics (tab.9).

Table 9. Equianalgesic ranges for loading doses of narcotics.

Loading doses	Alfentanil μg/kg	Fentanyl μg/kg	Sufentanil μg/kg
Small doses	20-40	6-12.5	1.25-2.5
Medium doses	40-80	12.5-25	2.5-5
High doses	80-450	25--150	5--30

The choice of the individual dose is highly dependant on the
post-operative needs for slow or rapid recovery of spontaneous
respiration. If high stress protection is required, high doses

are necessary, if medium or small doses are used, stable anesthesia may be obtained by the association of the potentiator
used in higher doses.

The optimal choice will depend on the possibilities of per-
and post-operative monitoring, type of patient and his pathology,
type and duration of surgery (depth, extent of the surgical
aggression). Finaly, the optimal narcotic dose for each patient
is the dose high enough to saveguard all the advantages of opiate
anesthesia and low enough to avoid the post-operative recovery
problems.

3.2. Monitoring

3.2.1. Clinical methods. Continuous observation of arterial
blood pressure, heart rate, hyperemia of the sclerae, lacrimation,
capillary oozing and diuresis, give a good indication regarding
adequateness of the NLA depth.

3.2.2. Electronic methods. In our opinion, the continuous trend
recording of the width of the peripherical pulse wave, associated
with the digital T° and the capnogram,possibly extended to the
thermal index of the peripheral circulation (TIPC),provides
the most reliable and earliest information about insufficient
stress protection during NLA.

3.2.3. Biochemical methods. Changes in plasma cortisol, ACTH,
GH, ADH, PRA, insulin, glucagon, glucose and urinary catecholamines and prostaglandines provide objective,but late,informations
regarding stress protection during different NLA techniques.
Personal investigations in this field will be discussed.

3.3. Choice of narcotic

After intensive investigations of the clinical possibilities

of alfentanil, sufentanil and lofentanil, we have for daily
practice turned back to fentanyl. It is used mostly in medium
IV loading doses of 12.5-25 µg/kg, associated with a potentiator-
corrector (62).

Alfentanil is mainly used for short interventions (40-160
µg/kg). Sufentanil, in relatively high doses (10-20 µg/kg), is
reserved for thoracic and major cardiovascular surgery.

Lofentanil is no longer in use in our clinic.

3.4. Intravenous infusions of narcotics

Continuous infusion of fentanyl or alfentanil, installed
after the administration of the loading dose of the same
substance, and supplemented by bolus injections as clinically
indicated, provide definite advantages compared to the common
practice of rapidly administering large IV doses of the opiate
for induction and maintenance of anesthesia (tab.10).

Table 10.Continuous infusion of narcotic : 3 step technique.

	Step 1 Loading dose µg/kg	Step 2 Continuous infusion 1th hour . 2-3th hour µg/kg/min		Step 3 Small bolus ★ µg/kg
-Fentanyl or -Alfentanil	10-20 40-80	0.10-0.15 1.0 -1.5	0.05-0.10 0.5 -1.0	2 8
★ for correction as clinically indicated				

With continuous infusion, higher stability of anesthesia is
obtained with a relatively lower total amount of narcotic. It can
be admitted that in doing so, the drug wasted in silent deposits
is reduced and the obtained CNS opiate levels are higher.
Therefore, the risk of remorphinisation or late recovery is low.

Nevertheless,fixed infusion rates have little place in clinical

practice because too great individual variations in sensibility
and catabolism of the opiates exist. For long lasting interventions the initial infusion rate is mostly followed by a slower
infusion from the 2th and 3th hour of surgery forth.

3.5. Choice of the potentiator corrector

Droperidol (0.25 -0.30 mg/kg) is still used for NLA by some
of our anesthesists.

Midazolam (0.2 mg/kg) is perhaps a better choice. Less side
effects are noted and amnesia is better guaranteed. No changes
have been observed in the hemodynamic variables currently
measured in our patients (31).

Etomidate (0.3 mg/kg) has our preference, compared to thiopentone. It allows a rapid reflex free induction. This dose is
not repeated during anesthesia (63).

Nitrous oxide. The addition of N20 to supplement fentanyl
anesthesia may not be as depressing as was previously believed.
If left ventricular function of the patient is good, no significant hemodynamic changes are seen, although the decrease in
cardiac index reach only a modest 13% (64). The addition of N20
70% to fentanyl, has no troublesome effects (65).

3.6. "Stress free" NLA ?

Adverse effects resulting from occasional and transient reflex
hyperactivity of the autonomic nervous system may not be very
troublesome. Persistant hyperactivity, however, must always be
prevented.

With the aid of careful monitoring and with the use of sufficiently high doses of the selected analgesia and neurolepsis
compounds, it is possible to obtain a near "stress free" NLA

during the per-operative period. In most cases however, this
protection does not persist long enough during the post-
operative period.

4. NLA TO MORROW

NLA research goes further in two directions:

- higher controlability of anesthesia, during the per-
operative period, using new compounds,

- broader protection of the patient during the perioperative period, with the help of long acting products.

4.1. New compounds

4.1.1. Analgesics. We now have at our disposal a wide
range of safe, potent, and specific substances with rapid or slow
onset, short or long duration of action. Their adaptation
to all types of surgical interventions is possible. The aim to
find potent analgesics without respiratory depression is still
an important research tool, but at the moment no solution is
in sight.

4.1.2. Neurolepsis. The ideal potentiator-corrector of the
narcotic is at yet not synthetised. There is still a need for a
more rapid and short acting product with adaptation possibilities to the individual basal tonus of the autonomic nervous
system.

The new antiserotonin compounds : ketanserin and butanserin
seem to offer new possibilities bringing us nearer to the goal
(see second lecture).

4.2. New concept : long acting protectors

Wide variation in individual sensitivity for nociceptive
stimuli and for sympathetic reactivity are responsible for drug

resistance and insufficient suppression of stress reactions during and after anesthesia. Activation of neurotransmission, by the neuromodulators: histamine, serotonin, catecholamines and prostaglandines are the underlying mechanisms for hyperactivity, unstable anesthesia and need for high doses of anesthesic drugs.

The use of safe, potent long lasting substances of the group of antihistaminics, antiserotonins, antiprostaglandines and/or calcium entry blockers, may offer the opportunity of stabilising neurotransmission on a lower level for a long time before, during, and after anesthesia. Reduction of the per-operative narcotic doses, reduction of the side effects and more comfort for the patient can perhaps be gained in this way (see second lecture).

REFERENCES

1. De Castro J, Mundeleer P. 1979. Anesthésie sans sommeil, neuroleptanalgésie. Acta Chir Belgica,7,689-691.
2. Laborit H. 1954. Réactions organiques à l'agression et choc. ed Masson,Paris.
3. Janssen P, Jagenau A. 1959. J Med Pharm Chem 1,105.
4. De Castro J, Mundeleer P. 1959. La neuroleptanalgésie, nouvelle technique d'anesthésie IV non barbiturique. Anesth Analg Réan (Fr),16,5,1022.
5. De Castro J, Mundeleer P. 1982. Die Neuroletpanalgesia, Auswahl der Preparate Bedeutung der Analgesie und der Neurolepsie. Anaesthesist, 11,1,10,1982.
6. Janssen P .1962.A review of the chemical features associated with strong morphine like activity. Brit J Anaesth, 34,260.
7. Dobkin AB, Lee PKY. 1963. Neuroletpanalgesie. Br J Anaesthesia,35,694.
8. Gemperle M. 1964. Medikamentoese Herabsetsung der Sauerstoffaufname durch Neuroleptanalgesie. Anaesthesist,13,181.
9. Nilsson E, Ingvar DH. 1965. Cerebral blood flow during neuroleptanalgesia. Acta Anaesth Scand,10,47.
10. Corsen G, Domino EF. 1964. Neuroleptanalgesia and anesthesia. Anesth analg, 43,748.
11. De Castro J, Mundeleer P. 1961. Neuroleptanalgesia and its problems,symposium, Royal Soc Med,London 24 may .
12. De Castro J. 1976. Practical applications and limitations of analgesic anesthesia.Acta Anesth Belgica ,3,107-128.

13. De Castro J. 1976. Les limites de l'anesthésie
    analgésique pure. Ann Anesth Fr,17,9,1071.
14. Vourc'h G et al.1971. Les analgésiques et la douleur
    ed Masson,Paris,225-282,418-461.
15. Gemperle M. 1970. La neuroleptanalgésie,ed Hans Huber,
    Bern.
16. Henschel WF. 1972. Neuroleptanagesie.ed Schattauer Verlag
    Stuttgart.
17. De Castro J, Van de Water A, Wouters L et al.1979.
    Comparative study of cardiovascular,neurological and
    metabolic side effects of eight narcotics in dogs.
    Acta Anesth Belgica,30,5-99.
18. Walley DG.1980. Oxygen and high dose fentanyl for
    aorto coronary bypass surgery.Meeting of 21 june,
    Can Anaesth Soc.
19. de Lange S,Stanley TH,Boscoe MJ et al.1983. Catecholamine
    and cortisol responses to high dose sufentanil-02 and
    alfentanil-02 anesthesia during coronary artery surgery,
    Canad anaesth soc J.30,248-254.
20. Ausems ME, Hug CCJr, de Lange S. 1983. Variable rate
    infusion of alfentanil as a supplement to nitrous oxide
    anesthesia for general surgery.Anesth and Analg,62,982-986.
21. Edde RR. 1981.Hemodynamic changes prior to and after sterno-
    tomy in patients anesthetized with high dose fentanyl.
    Anesthesiology,55,444-446.
22. De Castro J, Andrieu S, Boogaerts J.1982. Buprenorphine.
    Ars Medici,New Drug Series N°1. ed Kluwer,Antwerpen.
23. De Castro J, Andrieu S. 1983. New trends in neuroleptanalgesia
    Ars Medici,Congress Series 2, ed Kluwer Antwerpen.
24. De Castro J,Hoerig C. 1981. Die Pharmakokinetik von Fentanyl und
    deren Konsequenzen fuer Atemdepression und Remorphinisierung
    bei der analgetischen Anaesthesie.Anaesth Intensive Med,
    22,190-198.
25. De Castro J,Mundeleer P. 1962. NLA pratique.Agressologie,
    3 S29.
26. De Castro J. 1972. Contribution à l'étude de la pharmacologie
    clinique des analgésiques centraux:analyse de certaines actions
    du fentanyl utilisé à hautes doses en anesthésie et en
    réanimation. Thèse d'agrégation ULB Bruxelles .
27. De Castro J,Lecron L. 1973. Les analgésiques et l'anesthésie
    analgésique, Utilisation des morphiniques en anesthésie
    ed Arnette,Paris ,p255-281.
28. De Castro J Mundeleer P. 1962. L'aneurine,un anesthésique
    complèt;Agressologie,3,S127.
29. De Castro J Valenti F. 1968. La sinaptanalgesia,technica attuale
    Acta Anaesthesiologica;XIX,supl 1,39-53.
30. De Castro J,Lecron L. 1973. Ataranalgesie with flunitrazepam
    and fentanyl.Proc 5th world congress of anesth ,Kyoto,
    ed Excerpta Medica p184.
31. De Castro J et al. 1981. Etude du midazolam comme inducteur,
    correcteur et potentialisateur d'une anesthésie analgésique
    à base d'alfentanil.Drug Res,31,(II), 2251-2254.
32. De Castro J 1982. Autonomous nervous system hyperactivity
    during alfentanil-labetalol analgésic anesthésia.
    6th Eur Congress of Anaesth, ed Academic Press p435.

33. De Castro J 1982. Twenty five years of NLA,concepts,evolution
    actual trends.Int congress, history of anaesthesia,
    Eramus University,Rotterdam.
34. De Castro J. 1970. Utilisation per-anesthésique d'analgésiques
    à forte doses.Symposium anesthésie vigile,Ostende 1969,
    ed Ars Medici Nivelles et Masson Paris,1,4,38-85.
35. Bailey P, Gerbode F, Garlington L. 1958. An anesthetic technique
    for cardiac surgery which utilizes 100% oxygen as the only
    inhalant. Archives of Surgery ,76,437-440.
36. Lowenstein E, Hallowell P, Levine F et al. 1969.Cardiovascular
    response to large doses of intravenous morphine in man.
    New England J of medicine,281,1389-1393.
37. Lowenstein E. 1971. Morphine anesthesia,a perspective,
    Anesthesiology,35,563-565.
38. Hasbrouck JD. 1970. Morphin anesthesia for open-heart surgery
    Annals of thoracic surgery,10,363-369.
39. Defazio CA, Chen P. 1971. The influence of morphine on
    excess lactate production.Anesth Analg,50,2,211.
40. Eisenberg L, Kavan AM. 1971. Neuroleptanalgesia with
    diazepam morphine in poor risk surgical patients.
    Canad Anaesth Soc J, 18,4,465469.
41. Arens JF, Benbow BP,Oschner JL. 1972. Morphine anesthesia
    for aorto-coronary bypass procedures. Anesth and Analg
    51,901-907.
42. Stanley TH, Gray, NH Stanford W, et al.1973.The effects of
    high dose morphine on fluid and blood requirements in open
    heart surgery. Anesthesiology,38,536-541.
43. Stoelting RK, Gibbs PS, Cresser CW, et al. 1975. Hemodynamic
    and ventilatory responses to fentanyl,fentanyl-droperidol,
    and nitrous oxide in patients with acquired valvular
    disease.Anesthesiology,42,319-324.
44. Wong KC. 1983. Narcotics are not expected to produce
    unconsciousness and amnesia. Anesth and Analg 62,625-626.
45. McDermott RW, Stanley TH. 1974. The cardiovascular
    effects of low concentration of nitrous oxide during morphine
    anesthesia.Anesthesiology.41,89-91.
46. Bennett GM, Loeser EA, Stanley TH. 1977. Cardiovascular
    effects of scopolamine during morphine-oxygen and
    morphine-nitrous oxide-oxygen anesthesia in man.
    Anesthesology.46,225.
47. Grell FL, Kooms RA. 1970. Fentanyl in Anesthesia.
    Anesth and Analg. 49,523.
48. Liu WS, Bidawai AV, Stanley TH et al. 1976a. The cardio-
    vascular effects of diazepam and pancuronium during fentanyl
    and oxygen anesthesia. Cand Anaesth Soc J 23,395-403.
49. Stanley TH, Webster LR. 1978. Anesthetic requirements
    and cardiovascular effects of fentanyl-oxygen and
    fentanyl-diazepam-oxygen anesthesia in man. Anesth and Analg
    57,411-416.
50. Stanley TH,Philbin DM, Coggins CH. 1979. Fentanyl-oxygen
    anesthesia for coronary artery surgery,cardiovascular
    and hormonal responses. Canad Anaesth Soc J.26,168-172.
51. Liu WS, Bidawi AV, Stanley TH et al.1976b. Cardiovascular
    dynamics after large doses of fentnyl plus N20 in the dog.
    Anesth and Analg. 55,168-172.

52. Stanley TH, Berman L, Green O et al.1980. Plasma catecho-
    lamine and cortisol responses to fentanyl-oxygen anesthesia
    for coronary artery operations. Anesthesiology. 53,250-253.
53. de Lange S, Stanley TH, Boscoe MJ. 1980. Fentanyl-oxygen
    anesthesia,comparison of anesthetic requirements and
    cardiovascular responses in Salt Lake City and Leiden,Holland.
    Abstracts 7th world Congress of anesthesiology,Hamburg,FRG p313.
54. Kentor ML, Schwalb AJ, Lieberman RW. 1980. Rapid high doses
    fentanyl induction for CABG. Anesthesiology.53,S95.
55. Comstock MK, Carter JG, Moyer JR,et al. 1981. Rigidity and
    hypercarbia associated with high dose fentanyl induction
    of anesthesia. Anesth and Analg .60,362-363.
56. Hilgenberg JC.1981. Intraoperative awareness during high dose
    fentanyl-oxygen anesthesia. Anesthesiology.54,341-343.
57. Hug CC Jr. 1982. New narcotic analgesics and antagonists.
    Seminars in anesthesia 1,14-40.
58. Moldenhauer CC Hugh CC jr. 1982.Continuous infusion of
    fentanyl for cardiac surgery. Anesth and Analg 61,S206.
59. Sonntag H, Larsen R, Hilkifer O et al. 1982. Myocardial
    blood flow and oxygen consumption during high-dose
    fentanyl anesthesia in patients with coronary artery
    disease.Anesthesiology. 56,417-422.
60. De Castro J. 1974. Utilisation de naloxone après anesthésie
    analgésique.4th Eur.Congress of anesthesiology,Madrid,
    Excerpta Medica, Congress Series 330,p129.
61. De Castro J, Andrieu S. 1981. Is the use of high doses of
    morphinomimetic drugs justified during surgery?
    Post Graduate Course , 13th int meeting of anesthesiology
    ed Arnette Paris 119-133.
62. De Castro J. 1977. Analgesic anesthesia with alfentanil a new
    short acting morphinomimetic (first clinical trials)
    Unpublished Report , Janssen Pharmaceutica.
63. De Castro J, Mattez J. 1978. Use of alfentanil combined with
    etomidate. 5th Eur congress of anesthesiology ,Paris
    Excerpta medica,congress series 452,p259.
64. Balasaraswathi K,Kumur P, Rao TLK et al.1981. Left ventricular
    end diastolic pressure (LVEDP) as an index for nitrous
    oxide use during coronary artery surgery.Anesthesiology,
    55,708-7095.
65. Michaels I, Kay H, Barash P.1982. Does nitrous oxide or
    a reduced FiO2 alter hemodynamic function during high
    dose fentanyl anesthesia? Anesthesiology,57,A44.
66. Janssen P.1981. Potent,new analgesics,tailor made for different
    purposes.Janssen Research News,2,2-15.

THE NEW SEDATIVE/HYPNOTICS

ROBERT J. FRAGEN, M.D.

At the time of this meeting there are three new hypnotic
drugs that have either been approved for general use or are
undergoing studies in this country. Their pharmacology and
proposed uses in anesthesiology are described.

1. ETOMIDATE

Etomidate was introduced by Paul Janssen in Belgium in 1971
and was approved in this country about two years ago. A carboxy-
lated imidazole derivative [(R)- (+)-ethyo-1-(1-phenylethyl)-
1H-imidazole-5 carboxylate], 20 mg of etomidate (Amidate) is
dissolved in 10 ml of propylene glycol. It is stable in solution
and has a wide margin of safety in animals. The LD_{50}/ED_{50} is
25.4 which is about six times greater than that of thiopental
and twice that of methohexital. The recommended dose of 0.3
mg/kg acts in one arm-brain circulation time to produce a 3-5
minute period of unconsciousness. The duration of action can
be increased by increasing the initial dose or by giving additional doses. Doubling the dose doubles the sleep time.

Pharmacokinetic studies show that etomidate's short duration
of action is due to redistribution (tissue uptake) and hydrolysis
of the ester group in the liver. The volume of distribution,
clearance and elimination half-life of etomidate, thiopental,
methohexital and the other two new drugs are compared in the
table. Urinary excretion accounts for 87% of the drug and biliary
excretion for the rest. Etomidate is 75% protein bound and its
metabolites are inactive.

Etomidate decreases intracranial pressure, cerebral blood
flow and the cerebral metabolic rate for oxygen. Etomidate and
thiopental cause similar EEG changes. Cortical seizure activity

is absent during myoclonus, a possible induction side effect
of etomidate. Etomidate can be used safely in neurosurgery and
cerebral protection studies are encouraging.

Etomidate causes less respiratory depression than thiopental.
The respiratory rate and depth first increase slightly, but then
both decrease with an occasional short period of apnea. Those
who use etomidate should be prepared to assist ventilation.
Etomidate causes no histamine release and is safe to use in
patients with bronchoconstrictive disease.

Etomidate's forte is the absence of cardiovascular depression
when used to induce general anesthesia. Studies in patients
with cardiovascular disease and in healthy patients showed that
cardiovascular measurements changed little from control values
and one study suggested that etomidate may have a mild coronary
vasodilating effect.

Etomidate lowers plasma cortisol and aldosterone by an adrenal
cortical effect. This is probably of no serious consequence
in most patients but will prevent etomidate's use by continuous
long-term infusion. It is not toxic to the liver or kidney.

The negative aspects of etomidate's use are induction side
effects - pain on injection and myoclonia, occasional cough or
hiccough, and nausea and vomiting. Pretreatment with a narcotic
and slow injection into a large vein through a rapidly running
i.v. infusion minimize pain on injection and myoclonus. Nausea
and vomiting are seen mainly after short procedures.

Etomidate will probably be restricted to special situations
because of the above side effects and its high cost compared
to thiopental. These special situations would include patients
with a compromised cardiovascular system or those with broncho-
spastic disease.

2. MIDAZOLAM

Midazolam is a unique benzodiazepine because its salts are
water soluble and the drug can be injected i.v. or i.m. without
the irritation caused by the organic solvents of other benzodiazepines. It has either recently been approved for general
use as an anesthetic induction agent, i.v. sedative and i.m.

premedicant or is about to get FDA approval. Midazolam (Versed), introduced by Walser and Freyer in 1975, has been under investigation for 10 years by Hoffman-LaRoche, Inc. It comes in a multiple dose vial of 10 ml containing 5 mg/ml buffered to a pH of 3.5. At this pH, its benzodiazepine ring is open and the compound is water soluble. When injected into the body, the ring closes, it becomes lipid soluble and rapidly crosses the blood-brain barrier to produce its CNS effects.

Depending upon the dose injected, midazolam causes typical benzodiazepine characteristics: anxiolysis; hypnosis; anterograde amnesia (lack of recall); anticonvulsant properties; and muscle relaxation. It is shorter acting than other benzodiazepines and has a shorter half-life than thiopental when used for anesthetic induction. Midazolam is 96% protein bound and if its three metabolites are active, they don't prolong the action of the parent compound. Midazolam is metabolized in the liver and excreted by the kidney. The oral form of the drug undergoes significant first-pass metabolism in the liver and has a bioavailability of 44%. Bioavailability i.m. is over 90%.

Suggested doses are 0.2 mg/kg for anesthetic induction, titration of 0.05 mg/kg doses to the endpoint of slurred speech for i.v. sedation, and 0.07-0.08 mg/kg for i.m. premedication. Older men are more sensitive to its effects and more variability in response occurs in young, unpremedicated patients than occurs with thiopental.

Midazolam causes minimal cardiorespiratory depression. It produces a dose-related respiratory depression which can lead to a short-lived apnea. It doesn't alter airway mechanics but has a more prolonged effect in patients with COPD than does thiopental.

Mild cardiovascular effects include hypotension (usually about 10% decrease), decreased systemic vascular resistance and decreased left ventricular stroke work index. A mild compensatory increase in heart rate is sometimes seen. Thus, it can be given safely to normovolemic patients with heart disease but may cause unwanted hypotension in hypovolemic patients or those who start with a high vascular tone.

Midazolam's forte will be its lack of tissue irritation for
an injectable benzodiazepine, relatively short duration of effect
and strong amnesic effect. It will be used where injectable
diazepam is now used. It will be used to induce general anesthesia when a slow, pleasant induction is desired, as an i.v.
sedative during local and regional anesthesia or for diagnostic
procedures, and as an i.m. premedicant when anesthetic induction
will occur within 40 minutes.

3. DIPRIVAN

Currently under investigation, Diprivan is 2,6 diisopropyl
phenol dissolved in an emulsion, a duck-egg lecithin (intralipid-
type substance). It is a stable 1% solution containing 10 mg/ml
in a 15 ml ampule. Diprivan was originally dissolved in cremophor El by ICI in England but cremophor El is an unacceptable
solvent in this country because it causes anaphylactoid reactions
in susceptible individuals.

Diprivan has a short half-life (table) and is 90% protein
bound. It is metabolized in the liver and excreted by the kidney. Metabolites are inactive. It is a pure hypnotic and has
no known analgesic properties. A 2.5 mg/kg dose produces a 3-5
minute period of unconsciousness in one arm-brain circulation
time. Sleep time is linearly related to the dose. Patients,
once awake, usually stay awake and become clear-headed earlier
than with other induction agents.

Diprivan produces a dose-related respiratory depression including a brief period of apnea. Cardiovascular depression re-
sembles that produced by thiopental and is likely to be greater
in patients with a high vascular tone at the time of induction.
Diprivan depresses blood pressure (15-20%), stroke volume, systemic vascular resistance and left ventricular stroke work index.
Heart rate is usually increased resulting in an unchanged cardiac
output. By five minutes after injection, the cardiovascular
and respiratory measurements have usually returned to control
values.

One side effect is pain on injection, the severity of which
depends upon the size of the vein into which it is injected and

the prior administration of a narcotic. Very mild excitatory effects, i.e. involuntary movements, cough or hiccough are occasionally seen, especially in unpremedicated patients. The incidence of nausea and vomiting is low.

Diprivan will be under investigation for at least another two years. Because of its short duration of action and lack of hangover, it will be used for anesthetic induction for out-patient surgery and for short inpatient procedures.

TABLE. Mean pharmacokinetic calculations

Name of drug	Vd (L/kg)	Cl_{elim} (ml/min)	$t\frac{1}{2}\beta$ (hr)
Thiopental	1.6	144	6.2
Methohexital	1.1	825	1.6
Etomidate	4.5	740	4.6
Midazolam	1.8	265	1.3-2.4
Diprivan	4.5	3454	1.0

Vd = apparent volume of distribution, Cl_{elim} = total body clearance, and $t\frac{1}{2}\beta$ = elimination half-life.

REFERENCES

ETOMIDATE

1. Fragen RJ, Shanks CA, Molteni A, Avram MJ: Effects of etomidate on hormonal responses to surgical stress. Anesthesiology (in press).
2. Giese JL, Stanley TH: Etomidate: A new intravenous anesthetic induction agent. Pharmacotherapy 3: 251-258, 1983.
3. Kettler D, Sonntag H, Donath D et al.: Hamodynamik, myokardmechanik, sauerstoffbedarf und sauerstoffversorgung des menshlichen herzens unter nardoseinleitung mit etomidate. Anaesthesist 23: 116-121, 1974.
4. Moss E, Powell D, Gibson RM, McDowall DG: Effect of etomidate on intracranial pressure and cerebral perfusion pressure. Br J Anaesth 51: 347-352, 1979.

MIDAZOLAM

1. Connor JT, Katz RL, Pagano RR, Graham CW: RO 21-3981 for intravenous surgical premedication and induction of anesthesia. Anesth Analg 57: 1-5, 1978.
2. Forster A, Gardaz JP, Suter PM, Gemperle M: Respiratory depression by midazolam and diazepam. Anesthesiology 53: 494-497, 1980.

48

3. Fragen RJ, Funk DI, Avram MJ et al.: Midazolam versus hydroxyzine as intramuscular premedicants. Can Anaesth Soc J 30: 136-141, 1983.
4. Fragen RJ, Gahl F, Caldwell N: A water-soluble benzodiazepine, RO 21-3981, for induction of anesthesia. Anesthesiology 49: 41-43, 1978.
5. Greenblatt DJ, Abernethy DR, Locniskar A et al.: Effect of age, gender, and obesity of midazolam kinetics. Anesthesiology (in press).
6. Gross JB, Zebrowski ME, Carel WD et al.: Time course of ventilatory depression after thiopental and midazolam in normal subjects and in patients with chronic obstructive pulmonary disease. Anesthesiology 58: 540-544, 1983.
7. Hanno PM, Wein AJ: Anesthetic techniques for cystoscopy in men. J Urol 130: 1070-1072, 1983.
8. Lebowitz PW, Cote ME, Daniels AL et al.: Cardiovascular effects of midazolam and thiopentone for induction of anaesthesia in ill surgical patients. Can Anaesth Soc J 30: 19-23, 1983.
9. Magni VC, Frost RZ, Leung JWC, Cotton PB: A randomized comparison of midazolam and diazepam for sedation in upper gastrointestinal endoscopy. Br J Anaesth 55: 1095-1101, 1983.
10. Pieri L: Preclinical pharmacology of midazolam. Br J Clin Pharmacol 16: 17s-27s, 1983.
11. Reves JG, Vinik R, Hirschfield AM et al.: Midazolam compared with thiopentone as a hypnotic component in balanced anaesthesia: A randomized, double-blind study. Can Anaesth Soc J 26: 42-49, 1979.
12. Samuelson PN, Reves JG, Kouchoukos NT et al.: Hemodynamic responses to anesthetic induction with midazolam or diazepam in patients in ischemic heart disease. Anesth Analg 60: 802-809, 1981.

DIPRIVAN

1. Adam HK, Briggs LP, Bahar M et al.: Pharmacokinetic evaluation of ICI 35,868 in man. Br J Anaesth 55: 97-102, 1983.
2. Prys-Roberts C, Davies JR, Calverly RK, Goodman NW: Hemodynamic effects of infusions of diisopropyl phenol (ICI 35,868) during nitrous oxide anaesthesia in man. Br J Anaesth 55: 105-111, 1983.

NEW COMPOUNDS AND NEW SUPPLEMENTS FOR ANESTHESIA.

J.DE CASTRO

1. NEW COMPOUNDS FOR ANESTHESIA.

1.1. Narcotics.

Fentanyl was first synthetised in 1960 (1),twenty five years
of experience of this drug in the neuroleptanagesia (NLA) has
only increased its wide spread use. In an attempt to overcome
fentanyl limitations (chest rigidity,insufficient stress
protection, prolonged respiratory depression), derivatives of
fentanyl have been synthetised with higher analgesic potency,
faster onset and shorter duration of action (tab.1-2-3)

Table 1. Fentanyl and its analogues, first part (2).

Drugs	Synthesis (Janssen pharma.)	Clinical investigation	Release in Belgium	Lowest ED 50 mg/kg*	Safety margin
Fentanyl	1960	1960	1962	0.011	277
Carfentanil	1974	-	-	0.00034	10000
Sufentanil	1974	1975	1980	0.00071	25211
Lofentanil	1975	1975	-	0.00059	112
Alfentanil	1976	1976	1983	0.044	1080
* in animals, - = no informations					

Table 2. Fentanyl and its analogues, second part (3).

Drugs	Dose µg/kg	t1/2π min	t1/2α min	t1/2β min	VD L/kg	CL mL/kg/min
Fentanyl	6.4	1.7	13.4	219	4.0	12.7
Carfentanil	-	-	-	-	-	-
Sufentanil	5	0.7	13.7	149	2.5	11.3
Lofentanil	-	-	-	-	-	-
Alfentanil	50	1.3	9.4	94	1.0⁻	7.6

Table 3. Fentanyl and its analogues, third part (4).

Drugs	Onset IV activity min	Peak activity after min	Duration plain activity h	Duration rest activity h
Alfentanil	1/4	3	1/2	1/2-3/4
Fentanyl	1/2	6	1	1-2
Sufentanil	1/4	5	3/4	3/4-1
Lofentanil	20	60	8	14-16
Carfentanil	-	-	-	-

1.1.1. <u>Alfentanil</u>. Alfentanil is a pure fentanyl like narcotic in all its pharmacological characteristics, including clinical efficacy, drug interactions and side effects (5). Its particular pharmacokinetic profile explains certain differences.

It has the fastest onset and the shortest duration effect of any opioid. It can be used as a compound of anesthesia for short surgical procedures as well as for major surgery. Combined with etomidate,it can provide appropriate anesthesia for minor surgery in outpatients (6)

The most efficient method for its administration is a three step technique with an initial IV loading dose 40-80 μg/kg followed by an intravenous infusion of 1.0-1.5 μg/kg/min supple-mented as needed by small IV bolus doses 5.0-10 μg/kg. While there is an accumulation of alfentanil after repeated doses or during continuous infusion, patients will still recover more rapidly than after other narcotics. This is to be expected in view of its shorter elimination half time (7).

Professor Rosow will present in this session more detailed information about this attractive compound.

1.1.2. <u>Sufentanil</u>. Sufentanil is 5-10 X more potent than fentanyl as an analgesic. In qualitative terms, the effects of the compound on the respiratory system, cardiovascular system, and CNS, are very similar to those of fentanyl. According to our investigations, the only qualitative difference between the two products, lies in the possibility of providing a deeper stress protection with sufentanil than with fentanyl (8a,8b). This opinion is not unanimously accepted by other investigators.

Low doses of sufentanil 1-2 µg/kg, provide no differences between the two drugs (9, 10, 11, 12). High doses, in the range of 15-30 µg/kg, on the contrary produce less hypertension and tachycardia during major surgical aggression (13,14,15). Sufentanil's greater ability to prevent elevations of plasma AD and GH during major interventions, suggests that it may be more effective than fentanyl in blocking hormonal stress responses (16, 17, 18). Nevertheless, Rosow (19) found, even with 30 µg/kg, no evidence that hemodynamic stability is better with sufentanil. More recent studies showed that sufentanil, like alfentanil, or fentanyl, are unable to abolish increases in catecholamines during cardio-pulmonary bypass (20, 21).

1.1.3. Lofentanil. As with sufentanil, lofentanil is an extremely potent, pure analgesic. In contrast to sufentanil and fentanyl it is exceptionaly long lasting. An IV dose of 0.7 µg/kg produces a respiratory depression lasting up to 48 hours (22).

The long duration of action appears to be due to a prolonged fixation of the drug to specific receptor sites rather than to pharmacokinetic properties or storage in silent deposits. The onset of action is slow. The clinical study of the compound is difficult because there is a very individual sensibility. The appropriate doses are not easy to evaluate. Above all the fear of drug interactions and overdose are constant problems with lofentanil. Even more, reversal of the lofentanil depression needs very high and repeated naloxone dose. Practical use of lofentanil is limited. However, for research, the product provides a powerful tool for studying of the opiate receptors.

1.1.4. Carfentanil. Carfentanil is the most potent narcotic investigated up to now. Onset and duration of action lies in the same order as that of sufentanil. Solubility and absorption through the mucosae is particularly high. The substance has attracted most interest for immobilization of a wide range of wild animals (23).

Stanley has demonstrated that the potency and solubility profile of carfentanil in dogs makes it a useful narcotic to administer as a nebulized mist and also for topical application to the nasal mucous membranes (24). In Europe, carfentanil is not released for clinical use .

Present place of the narcotics in NLA. We can say that, perhaps for people who had high expectations of the new compounds, there is a little disappointment. Chest rigidity, individual sensibility, lack of amnesia, insufficient stress protection, are the same drawbaks seen with the new products as with fentanyl. Nevertheless, the new products have, in a large way, broadened our knowledge of opiate receptors and opiate kinetics.

The place that the new narcotics can occupy in the anesthesiological armentarium is certainly becoming wider and more versatile. Above all, the risk of remorphinisation after alfentanil is very low, and indications are very great.

For all these reasons, in our opinion,fentanyl still remains

a good choice for current NLA. Minor interventions are best
served by alfentanil, while for major surgery, particularly
cardiac surgery, sufentanil or alfentanil may have preference.

One other logical option, justified for practical reasons, is
the selection of alfentanil for all surgical interventions.

1.3. New antiserotonins.

1.2.1. Ketanserin, pirenperone and butanserin. Since 1981
several new potent serotonin blockers have been synthetised
in the laboratories of Dr. Paul Janssen.

Common properties of these substances are high binding
affinity on the 5HT 2 receptors, no activity on the 5HT 1
receptors and, depending on the product, weak to high anti
alpha 1 adrenergic activity, anti alpha 2 adrenergic affinity,
anti H 1 activity and antidopamine activity (25) (Table 4).

Some compounds of this new group have only peripheral
activities. Others act both on the peripheral and central
nervous system.

Table 4. Receptor binding of the new antiserotonins (26),
(Kl nm-in vitro).

Receptors	New antiserotonins			Neuroleptics
	Ketanserin	Pirenperone	Butanserin	Droperidol
5HT 2	2.1	2.0	3.3	4.1
5HT 1	n.a.*	n.a.	n.a.	n.a.
H 1	10	14	55.0	2200
Alpha 1	10	6.8	0.1	0.8
Alpha 2	0	3.3	200.0	2600
Dopamine	220	16	63.0	0.8
AcCh-M	n.a.	n.a.	n.a.	n.a.

* n.a.=>10000   (Leysen 1982)

Several of these substances are now under clinical investigation in the field of vascular or psychiatric diseases.
It is well known that serotonin is increased in many pathological situations and also during major surgery. High serotonin plasma levels are responsible for drug resistance, peripheral vaso-constriction, increased platelet aggregation and indirect amplification of the excitatory effects of most neurotransmitter substances : adrenaline, noradrenaline, histamine, vasopressine etc..(27).

The similarities of these new antiserotonin products with the receptor binding properties of droperidol, have focused our attention on these drugs for their utilisation in anesthesia in association with, or without, narcotics. Table 4 compares the relative potency of the receptor binding of 3 antiserotonin compounds with those of droperidol (28).

Up to now we have investigated firstly in dogs and after in man, ketanserin, pirenperone and butanserin :three antiserotonins with important alphalytic properties and weak toxicity (the LD50 of ketanserin is, in mice, 40 mg/kg IV).They have been used alone, or in association with fentanyl or alfentanil (29,30,31).

With pirenperone, a compound active on the dopamine receptor, extrapyramidal symptoms have been observed and the clinical investigation with this product in anesthesia has now been abandoned.On the other hand,ketanserin and butanserin (weak antidopamine blockers), used in IV doses of 0.4 and 0.03 mg/kg respectively, have given promising results during their daily use for NLA for more than 4 years. Extrapyramidal symptoms have never been seen.The maximum total doses for the 2 products used in our investigation during clinical anesthesia, are respectively 250 and 5 mg/70kg, body weight.

The clinical properties of butanserin are very similar to those of ketanserin, but the product has, on a weight basis, a 20 X higher alphalytic potency and a somewhat shorter duration of action.

The name of "alphaleptanalgesia"(ALA) was proposed for the associated use of alphalytic drugs with a narcotic (32).

1.2.2. Alphaleptanalgesia.

 - Technique. The most satisfying ALA technique with butanserin or ketanserin is given in table 5.

Table 5. Alphaleptanalgesia technique with butanserin
          or ketanserin.

Drugs	Doses	Comment

Induction :
 - etomidate
 - fentanyl
    or
   alfentanil
 - pancuronium
	0.3 mg/kg
	10-15 μg/kg
	
	40-60 μg/kg
	0.06 mg/kg
		The 3 drugs are mixed together in 1 seringue for slow injection. *

Intubation		

Stabilisation
 - butanserin
    or
   ketanserin
	0.03 mg/kg
	
	0.4 mg/kg
		injection is only done after compensation of the circulating volume

Maintenance
 - fentanyl
    or
   alfentanil
 - N20/02
 - pancuronium
 - butanserin
    or
   ketanserin
	0.2 μg/kg/min
	
	1.0 μg/kg/min
	60/40%
	0.01 mg/kg
	0.015 mg/kg
	
	0.2 mg/kg
		continuous infusion
		
		(on demand)

* simultaneous injection of the 3 drugs avoid jerk movements, injection pain and chest rigidity		

- Results. Cardiovascular system. The simultaneous administration of the antiserotonin substances with the other anesthetic drugs for loading, may provide over important peripheral vasodilation and hypotension. For this reason the hypnotic, the narcotic and the muscle relaxant are injected simultaneously before the antiserotonin. It is necessary to have a small pause between the 2 administrations to allow the correction of circulating blood volume with a plasma expender.

The administration of the antiserotonin after the narcotic produces an important increase in the peripheral temperature, an important peripheral vasodilation,a rise in the venous capacitance, a decrease in the arterial pulmonary pressure, in blood pressure, in cardiac work, in $M\dot{V}O2$ and an important reduction of capillary oozing. The myocardium is not depressed and diuresis is exellent.

Endocrine system. A decrease in plasma cortisol, ACTH and GH with an increase in PL and PRA and stable aldosterone levels are seen during and after ALA.

Central nervous system. In the per-operative period, narcotic and muscle relaxant doses can be saved. In the post-operative period ,absence of important prolongation of the opiate depression or the curarizing effects, early spontaneous respiration, slight sedation, marked anxiolysis, and reduced motor activity are noted. Muscle hypotonia, dysphoria, catatonia, tremor, or involuntary movements, are not seen.

Side effects. Hypotension can be compensated by adjustment of the circulating volume. Reflex tachycardia can be neutralised by supplementary doses of the narcotic.

   - Discussion.   Advantages of ketanserin or butanserin,
used in combination with a strong narcotic for ALA are evidenced
by comparison with droperidol or midazolam (tab.6). During the
surgical intervention, the stress protection, provided by antiserotonin is higher. The potentiation of the narcotic is great
but has a shorter duration and post operative respiratory
depression seldom occurs.

Table 6 . General trends in the comparative properties of
         4 narcotic potentiators used for NLA.

	ketan-serin	butan-serin	mida-zolam	drope-ridol
Doses (mg/kg)	0.5-2	0.025-0.05	0.2	0.4
IV effects :rapid onset	+	+	+	+
duration (h)	2-3	1-2	4-6	6-12
Safety,efficiency	+	+	+	+
- Peroperative period				
Cardiovascular system :				
. contractility	=	=	=	=
. hypotension	+	+ +	=	+
. tachycardia	+	+	-	=
. TICP	↗↗	↗↗	↗	↗
. PVR	↘↘	↘↘	↘	↘
. capillary oozing	↘↘	↘↘	↘	=
Bronchospasticity			=	=
Psychism	=	=	drow.	indif.
Muscle tonus				/
Stress protection	+ +	+ +	+	+
Potentiation of narcotic	+	+	+ +	+
Potentiation of muscle relaxant	+	+	+ +	-
- Postoperative period				
Duration of potentiatio	short	short	long	long
Prolongation of narcotic respiratory depression	no	no	yes	yes
Risk of remorphinisation	-	-	+	+
Vigilance	sed.	sed.	draw.	sed.
Anxiolysis	+ +	+ +	+	-
Muscle tonus	norm.	norm.	hypot.	dyst.
Vomiting %	6	5	16	8
Stress protection	+ +	+ +	-	+
Return of pain (h)	2-4	2-3	1-2	2-5

↗ = increased,   ↘ = decreased, + = exist, - = no exist

A disadvantage of the antiserotonins is the reflex tachycardia seen in some cases and also the wide variability in individual sensibility; however, these drawbacks are encountered with all the compounds acting on the autonomic nervous system.

In resistant patients small doses of midazolam (0.1 mg/kg) may be added to the antiserotonin substance (33).

2. NEW SUPPLEMENTS FOR ANESTHESIA.

2.1. Peri-anesthesia (PA) : a new approach to anesthesia.
The rationale of PA can be summarized as follows.

2.1.1. Stress and pain problems in the peri-anesthesia period.

a) The premedication administred just before the surgical intervention has still many drawbacks :

- the time shedule of administration is often inappropriate,
- the doses have a poor flexibilty,
- the efficacity is rarely optimal, side effects may occur.

Its real mission to provide more comfort and more security to the patient and ease to allow a more stable anesthesia,is not always fulfilled.

b) General anesthesia by itself is,in daily practice, limited to either inhalation anesthesia or NLA performed with small or medium doses of a narcotic.

Analgesic anesthesia with high doses of opiates is reserved to the management of cardiac and thoracic surgery because of the prolonged post-operative respiratory depression (34,35).

During the per-operative period, inhalation anesthesia, and NLA with small or medium doses of narcotics,provide, insufficient stress protection.

c) Stress and pain after surgery continue to evade reliable

clinical management. Stress protection by narcotics is only
transient; no effect was demonstrated in the post-operative
period and nitrogen inbalance cannot be improved during the first
post-operative days (36,37).

It is clear that the two commonly used clinical techniques of
postoperative pain control: regional anesthesia or intermittent
injections of analgesic drugs are providing an inadequate
solution. Urgent improvement in postoperative pain managment
has been emphasised

d) Anaphylactic accidents (1/4000 cases) (38) and thromboembolic complications (1/200 cases) during and after anesthesia
and surgery are still serious(39).

All these problems await a really new approach to anesthesia.
The synthesis of specific, potent and long lasting new compounds
may, perhaps, offer new possibiliies and fill up the blanks.
These products may put the patient's organism on full resting
levels before, during and after surgery. They provide a more
intensive preparation for anesthesia and their benefical effects
may be displayed the whole peri-operative period.

2.1.2. Stress and pain responses,release mechanisms and
modulation of nociceptive stimuli. In the peripheral and central
neuroaxons and in the smooth vascular muscles, stress and pain
provide the activation and release of a series of neurotransmitter
substances.

Positive modulators, accentuate the transmission of nociceptive stimuli, a.o. histamine, kinins, serotonin, catecholamines,
prostaglandines (40,41).

Negative modulators, reduce the transmission of nociceptive

stimuli, a.o. endorphins, enkephalins, GABA (42).

The binding of these endohormones on the specific receptors in the membrane of nerve cells and smooth muscles cells, initiate either the intracellular activation of adenylcyclase or the guanylcyclase, according to positive or negative effects. In the first situation, AMPc and Ca2+ entry increase, producing excitation and contraction. In the second situation, CMPc and Ca2+ outflow increase, producing inhibition and relaxation (43).

During the pre- per- and post-operative periods, notwithstanding the use of depressive drugs, the activation of the positive neuromodulators goes frequently far beyond the inhibition of the negative neuromodulators, resulting in excessive response of most physiological systems: cardiovascular and hormonal hyperactivity, spasticity of the smooth muscles with peripheral, splanchnic and renal vasoconstriction, oliguria, capillary oozing, bronchoconstriction, increased need for anesthetics, agitation, anxiety, pain and restlessness, muscle rigidity, metabolic acidosis, platelet aggregation and anaphylactic manifestations.

2.1.3. Classical drugs for pain and stress protection.
Premedication, anesthesia, and postoperative medication, are not always able to restore the balance of neurotransmission, on a adequate and sufficiently low level.

The reasons for unsatisfactory results with the classical drugs (hypnotics, sedatives, tranquillisers, antihistamines, analgesics) are threefold :

a) Constant changes in the intensity of the stimuli,

b) Constant changes in the reactivity responses of the patient,

c) Fractionated administration of drugs with peak effects of relatively short duration.

2.1.4. Stress and pain protection by use of long lasting compounds. In the presence of the partially unsatisfactory results obtained with the techniques used up to now, we have formed the hypothesis that the pain and stress responses of the patient can be more easily stabilised by the use of slow and long lasting substances, inhibiting partially (but for a long period) the positive modulators of nociceptive stimuli transmission.It is mandatory that such treatment covers, the periods preceding, accompagning and following the surgical intervention.
For these reasons it is important that the compounds selected for PA have the following properties : wide margin of the clinical security index, high specificity, minimal side effects, slow onset, long duration, high oral bioavaliability, free of unwanted drug interactions, and active on the histamine, serotonin and/or Ca2+ entry receptors.

Such a treatment goes far beyond a simple premedication,it can be best called "peri-anesthesia" (PA). Beneficial effects of this therapy may consist of: sedation, anxiolysis, spasmolysis, analgesia, protection against allergic and thromboembolic complications.

These effects last long, from the evening before the intervention to the post-operative period. They can also be extended, if necessary, after the surgical intervention.
2.2.New compounds for PA.

Recently, Doctor Paul Janssen's laboratories have synthetised new compounds fitting well to the enumerated PA desiderata. We have selected: levocabastine, a new antihistamine (44);

ritanserin, a new antiserotonin (45,46); flunarizine,
lidoflazin, R 51469, three calcium entry blockers, synthetised
some years ago (47,48); R59655, a new prostaglandine inhibitor,
with thromboxane A2 synthetase blocking activity (49).

2.2.1. <u>Levocabastine</u>. Levocabastine is the most potent and most
specific antihistamine presently at our disposal:

- anti H 1 potency = astemizole X 65,
- lowest active dose = 2-3 ug/kg,
- duration of action of 10 ug/kg = 32 hours,
- LD 50/ED 50 is > 1,706,666. mg/kg IV in mice,
- peak activity by oral route is reached after 2 hours and
  plasma t $1/2\beta$= 32 hours,
- bioavaliability by mouth is > 100%,thus parenteral
  administration is needless.

The only side effect noted in man, after the administration
of the standard dose (0.5 mg tablet), was a slight sedation.
The pharmacological effects of the substance are limited to
a block of histamine release, protection against anaphylactic
shock and against allergic symptoms.

2.2.2. <u>Ritanserin</u>. Ritanserin is the most specific, the most
potent and the most long lasting compound among the 5HT 2 blockers
(tab.7). The anti 5HT 2 activity is 10 x more potent than that

Table 7. Comparative affinity of receptor binding of
         ketanserin and ritanserin (K1,nM)(46):

Drugs	5HT1	5HT2	H1	H2	α1	α2	DA	AcCh-M
- Ketanserin	n.a.	2.1	10	n.a.	10	n.a.	220	n.a.
- Ritanserin	n.a.	0.2	24	n.a.	35	60	22	n.a.

of ketanserin altough its antihistamine, antidopamine, anti alpha 1
activities are very weak. LD 50/ED 50 = 6370 mg/kg IV in mice.

In man, the useful orally dose is 10-20 mg. Peak effects are
reached after 1 h and plasma t $1/2\beta$ = 100 h. Bioavaliability, by
oral route, is 100%. The pharmacological properties are charac-
terised by marked anxiolysis, peripheral and central antiserotonin
effects, inhibition of hyperactivity of catecholamines, and of
other vasoactive substances.

2.2.3. Flunarizine, lidoflazine and R 51459. Flunarizine
(10 mg per os) has shown most interesting properties as a
protector against cerebral vascular spasms, hyperviscosity
of the blood and brain ischemia (50).

The cardioprotective effects of lidoflazine and R 51469 were
investigated in dogs and clinically in patients undergoing
aortocoronary bypass grafting.

In the pharmacologically pretreated group with lidoflazine
1.0 mg/kg p.o. LVSWI remained unalterated, the sarcolemna of the
myocardium was preserved; ATP, creatine phosphate and glycogen in
transmural LV biopsies taken before, cross clamping and after
cessation of cardiopulmonary bypass, remained unchanged. Calcium
accumulation in damaged mitochondria was absent. The preservation
of high energy phosphates was significantly better, compared to
the control group.

The results demonstrate that pretreatment with calcium entry
blockers, improves myocardial tolerance to ischemia in open heart
surgery (51).

2.2.4. R 59655 is the first specific thromboxane blocker.
However our requirement for substances with long lasting activity

has till now, not been resolved. New derivatives of this compound
are under investigation (52).

2.3. Practical application of PA.

Our clinical investigation in the field of PA has recently
started. The only drug combination studied at this moment is the
association of levocabastine and ritanserin. Oral doses of
respectively 0.5 and 20 mg are respectively given the evening
before the surgical intervention.

The anxiolytic effects of the combination are remarkable and
long lasting. The fentanyl doses are reduced by 50%. The cardiovascular hyperactivity is reduced in an important way. Awakening
is rapid, free of problems and without noticable respiratory
depression. Side effects before or after the anesthesia are not
seen. The required amount of analgesics during the first post-
operative day is minimal. Plasma cortisol is stable during and
after surgery.

Indications and formulae for PA: The proposed PA medication
is useful in the preparation of patients for classical general
anesthesia, analgesic anesthesia, neuroleptanalgesia and loco-
regional anesthesia.

Table 8. The objectives of peri-anesthesia.

Objectives	Pre-op period	Per-op period	Post-op period
- Patient comfort	↑	↑	↑
- Pain	↘	↘	↘
- Stress protection	↗	↗	↗
- Anaphylaxis	↘	↘	↘
- Thromboembolism	↘	↘	↘
- Amount of anesthetics		↘	↘
- Drug resistance		↘	
- Drug hypersensibility	↘	↘	↘
- Anesthesia stability		↗	
- Endocrine stress response	↘	↘	↘

Our experience with PA therapy is certainly still too limited
to allow any conclusion.Nevertheless the results, so far obtained,
indicate that the approach to the PA objectives (tab.8) is
promising. We are convinced that the PA research to day, forms
the basis of a rational clinical practice for tomorrow

REFERENCES

1. Janssen P, Eddy N et al. 1960. New chemical methods of
   increasing the analgesic activity of pethidine.
   J Med Pharm Chem, 2,31.
2. Janssen P . 1981. Janssen Research News, 2,2-15.
3. Janssen P. 1980. A fentanyl family of analgesics,sufentanil,
   alfentanil and lofentanil.Research report Janssen Pharmaceutica, sept.
4. Janssen P. 1982. Potent,new analgesics,tailor made,for
   different purposes. Acta anaesth Scand,26, 262-268.
5. Janssen P. 1981. Alfentanil,R39209,a potent extremely
   short acting and safe intravenous narcotic analgesic.
   Investigational new drug brochure,Janssen Pharmaceutica,
   sept.
6. Kay B. 1983. Alfentanil. Clinics in anesthesiology.
   1,1,143-146,1983.
7. De Castro J . 1977. Analgesic anesthesia with alfentanil
   a new short acting morphinomimetic (first clinical trials).
   Unpublished report,july 1977.
8a. De Castro J. 1976. Symposium : new agents and adjuvants drugs
   in anesthesia,6th World Congress of Anesthesiology,Mexico
   city ,ed SAC Charleroi 96-114.
8b. De Castro J, Mattez J. 1976. Le choix du curarisant dans
   differents types d'anesthésie analgésique à base de sufentanil.
   6th World Congress of Anesthesiology,Mexico city,ed SAC
   Charleroi 115-134.
9. Larsen R, Sonntag H, Schenck HD et al. 1980. Die Wirkungen
   von Sufentanil und Fentanyl auf haemodynamik,Coronardurch-
   blutung und myocardialen Metabolismus des Menschen.
   Anaesthetist,29,277-279.
10. Rolly G, Kay B,et al. 1979. A double blind comparison of high
   doses of fentanyl and sufentanil in man.Acta Anesth Belgica,
   30,297-254.
11. Dubois Primo J, De Wachter B et al. 1979. Analgesic anesthesia
   with fentanyl and sufentanil in coronary surgery.A double blind
   study,Acta Anesth Belgica,30,113-126.
12. Van de Walle J,Lauwers P,Adriaensen H. 1976.Double blind
   comparison of fentanyl and sufentanil.Acta Anesth Belgica,
   27,129-138.

66

13. De Lange S, Boscoe MJ, Stanley TH. 1982. Comparison of sufentanil- 02 and fentanyl-02 for coronary artery surgery, Anesthesiology,56,112-118.
14. Griesemer RW, Moldenhauwer CC, Hug CC. 1982. Sufentanil anesthesia for aortocoronary bypass surgery.Anesthesiology, 57,A48.
15. Sebel PS, Bovill JG.1982.Cardiovascular effect of sufentanil anesthesia. Anesth and Analg,61,115-119.
16. Arroyo JL,Nalda MA. 1976. Réponse sympathico-adrénergique et hypophysaire à différentes techniques d'anesthésie analgésique 6th World Congress,Mexico city,ed SAC Charleroi,140-144.
17. Bovill JG, Sebel PS, Fiolet JWT et al. 1983. The influence of sufentanil on endocrine and metabolic response to cardiac surgery.Anesth and Analg,62,391-397.
18. de Lange S, Boscoe MJ, Stanley TH, et al. 1982. Antidiuretic and grow hormone response during coronary artery surgery with sufentanil-oxygen anesthesia in man.Anesth and Analg, 61,434-438.
19. Rosow CE. 1983. Sufentanil vs fentanyl: I. Suppression hemodynamic responses. Anesthesiology, 59,3A ,A 323.
20. de Lange S, Boscoe MJ, Stanley TH, et al . 1982. Comparison of sufentanil-02 and fentanil-02 for coronary artery surgery. Anesthesiology, 56, 112-118.
21. Spriggs JM, Wynands JE,Whalley DG,et al. 1982. Fentanyl infusion anesthesia for aortocoronary bypass surgery:plama levels and hemodynamic response. Anesth and Analg,61, 972-978.
22. Leyssen JE, Niemegeers CJE, Stanley TH. 1980. In vivo narcotic effects and opiate receptor occupation; 7th World Congress of anesthesiology,Hamburg,Excerpta Medica,congress series,p287.
23. De Vos V. 1978. Immobilization of free-ranging wild animals using a new drug.Veterinary Record,103,4,64.
24. Port JD, Stanley TH. 1983. Topical narcotic anesthesia. Anesthesiology,59,3A,A325.
25. Van Neuten JM et al. 1981. Vascular activity of ketanserin. Arch Int Phamac Ther ,250,2,328-329.
26. Leysen JE, Awouters F, Kennis L, et al. 1981.receptor binding profile of R 41468,a novel antagonist at 5-HT2 receptors.Life Science,28,9,1115-1122.
27. Van Nueten JM,et al . 1982. Interaction between 5-HT and other vasoconstrictor substances in rabbit.Effect of ketanserin. Eur J Pharmacol (in press).
28. De Castro J. 1981. Ketanserin,stress and anesthesia.Workshop, stress and serotonin in animals and man.8 sept.Beerse.
29. De Castro J. 1982. Ketanserin,alfentanil infusion anesthesia for major surgery.6th Eur Congress of anesthesiology,London ed Academic Press p435.
30. De Castro J, Arroyo JL et al.1982. Endocrinal and metabolic changes produced by ketanserin-alfentanil analgesic anesthesia 6th Eur Congress of anesthesiology,London, ed Academic Press, p435.
31. De Castro J, Van de Water A, Xhonneux R.1982. Cardiac and hemodynamic effects of the combined administration of high doses of ketanserin and alfentanil in dogs. 6th Eur Congress of anesthesiology,ed Academic Press,p436.

32. De Castro J, Andrieu S. 1983.New trends in Neuroleptanalgesia
    Int.Symp. L'anesthesiologiste devant le probleme de la
    douleur,february,Mons Belgium,Ars Medici, Congress Series 2,
    ed M et I S.A.,Bruxelles,1-141.
33. De Castro J. 1983. De la neuroleptanalgésie vers l'alphalept-
    analgésie 29th Congres Fr d'anesthesiologie,Lille.
34. Bennett MRD, Adams AP. 1983. Postoperative respiratory compli-
    cations of opiates. Clinics in anaesthesiology,1,1,41-56.
35. Moldenhauer CC, Hug CC. 1984. Use of narcotic analgesics as
    anesthsics.Clinics in anaesthesiology,2,1,107-138.
36. Walsh ES, Paterson JL. 1981. Effect of high dose fentanyl
    anesthesia on the metabolic and endocrine response to
    cardiac surgery. Br J Anaesth ,53,1155-1165.
37. Lowenstein E,Philbin DM.1983. Narcotic anaesthesia.
    Clinics in Anaesthesiology,1,1,5-15.
38. Rosow CE,Moss J, Philbin DM et al. 1983. Histamine release
    during morphine and fentanyl anesthesia.Anesthesiology,
    56,93-96.
39. Simpson PJ. 1984. Adverse reaction to IV Anaesthetic agents.
    Clinics in Anaesthesiology,2,1,185-202.
40. Gateau O .1983. Prostaglandines et douleur,modulation
    complexe de la nociception,Symp Int L'anesthésiologiste
    devant le probleme de la douleur,Mons,Belgium,Ars Medici,
    Congress series,3,1,23-44.
41. Vanhoutte PM,.1982. Effects of calcium entry blockers on
    Hypoxia. J of cerebral blood flow and metabolism,2 supl,
    S42-S44.
42. Ferreira SF. 1979. Site of analgesic action of aspirin-like
    drugs and opioids.Mechanisms of pain and analgesia compounds,
    ed Raven Press NY ,309-333.
43. Mayer SE. 1980. Neurohormonal transmission and the autonomic
    nervous system.Goodman and Gilman's The pharmacological
    basis of Therapeutics 6th ed McMillan Publ NY,p 56-90.48.
44. Janssen P. 1984. The first fully specific H 1 antagonist.
    Investigational New Drug Brochure 2th ed, march ,Janssen
    Pharmaceutica.
45. Ceulemans C et al. 1984. Serotonine blockade or benzo-
    diazepine what kind of anxiolysis. Abstract 14th CINP
    Congress,Florence,Italy.
46. Leysen JE,et al. 1983. Receptor binding profile of ritanserin.
    Preclinical Research Report. Janssen Pharmaceutica.
47. Vanhoutte PM, Van Nueten JM. 1982. Lidoflazine.New Drug
    Annual,ed Scriabin.
48. Flament W, Xhonneux R, Borgers M et al. 1982. Myocardial
    protection in open heart surgery ,R 51459 (in press)
49. De Clerck F, et al 1983. Platelet-vessel wall,interactions
    in hemostasis,implication of 5-hydroxytryptamine.
    Research Report,Janssen Pharmaceutica.
50. Reyntjens AJM. 1982. The clinical effects of two calcium
    entry blockers cinnarizine and flunarizine. Janssen
    Pharmaceutica,Investigational Report.
51. Flameng W, Daenen W, Bogers M,et al. 1981. Cardioprotective
    effects of lidoflazine during 1 hour normothermic global
    ischemia. Circulation64,796.
52. De Clerck F. 1984. Personal communication.

VERY POTENT COMPOUNDS AND NEW APPROACHS TO ANESTHESIA

THEODORE H. STANLEY, M.D.

The last 20 years have seen numerous developments in neurophysi-
ology and neuropharmacology.1-12 One of the most important of these,
which will undoubtedly have a significant impact on Anesthesiology,
is in the discipline of neurotransmission. It is now believed that
there are many neurotransmitters in the central nervous system (CNS)
that act at a variety of receptor sites and affect all forms of human
behavior. In addition, it is clear that many of the CNS neurotransmitters interact and/ or otherwise influence each other both qualita-
tively and quantitatively. As a result, chemists, developmental
pharmacologists and some research anesthesiologists, in conjunction
with a number of pharmaceutical companies and governmental agencies,
have been interested in the synthesis of new, extremely potent narcotic
analgesics, sedative/hypnotics, central peptide-like drugs and other
compounds which can influence CNS neurotransmitters. The objective of
this manuscript will be to discuss the rationale that has produced
research to develop very potent central acting compounds and has sec-
ondarily resulted in new techniques and approachs to anesthesia. Some
examples of the new drugs and how they will be administered will also
be addressed.

Why a very potent compound?

Laboratory animal and clinical experience with numerous classes of
compounds has suggested that as the potency of compounds increases, side
effects decrease.13-18 This is clearly seen in the evolution of the new
opioids. Older compounds like morphine, meperidine and alphaprodine are
relatively impotent and possessed of low therapeutic indeces or safety
margins (5-70) in rats and dogs. All of the new opioids such as carfentanil, lofentanil, alfentanil, sufentanil and other experimental compounds
(simply known by number) have much higher therapeutic indeces,

these vary from as low as 1000 to as high as 45,000.[14]* Compounds that
act at receptors like opioids, benzodiazepines, GABA receptor stimulators and other neurotransmitters should produce less side effects as
their potency increases because less drug is required and thus less action at sites, other than the receptor, are possible. That this may be
an advantage is now being seen in the design of even more specific receptor compounds, for example, the numerous receptor subtypes now described for the opioids (kappa, sigma, delta, mu_1, mu_2, and others).
[3,11,12,19] It has recently been suggested, that it is now possible
to produce profound analgesia with minimal or no respiratory effects
using new opioids that are specific for one or more of the opioid receptor subtypes.[3,19,20] Whether this is indeed true in man is still to be
confirmed, however, numerous animal studies suggest that it is possible.
Thus, the development of new compounds specific for the mu_1 receptor
(meptazimol) result only in analgesia and catalepsy.[3.20-23] In
contrast, other compounds specific for the mu_2 receptor result in
respiratory depression without analgesia.

High potency allows other fascinating applications of compounds.
Research in our laboratories has demonstrated that it is possible to
nebulize highly potent opioids and other psychic acting drugs (in closed
containers) and produce various degrees of analgesia, sedation and anesthesia.[24] The use of highly potent compounds in concentrated solutions
also allows transmucosal administration with reasonably rapid onset of
analgesia, sedation, and, if enough drug is given, anesthesia.[25] It
has recently become clear that it is also possible to apply very potent
drugs on the skin of animals and achieve varying degrees of analgesia
and/or anesthesia (Port JD, personal communication). The evolution of
these new techniques suggests that administration of anesthesia, as well
as the compounds used for anesthesia, may dramatically change in the
future. Imagine, for example, inducing anesthesia with a lollipop or
with a bandaid. Let us go one step further and make bandaids saturated
with very potent compounds that can produce a peak effect in a short
period of time, 10-30 minutes. It should be possible to vary the duration of activity, depending on the specific compounds, from a few minutes
to a few days. Since the compound's peak action could occur in a very

---

*Burns W and Turrell R, unpublished data

short period of time the bandaid could be removed at the time of peak effect; then the duration of action would simply depend on the unique pharmacokinetics of the compound in question. This could vary from a few hours, to a day or two or possibly a week or more.

Theoretically, transdermal applications avoid problems secondary to gastrointestinal absorption (variability of onset and/or duration, gastric irritation, gastric ulceration, etc.). In addition, onset of action and duration of activity should be more predictable, blood and brain concentrations more constant and, depending upon the compounds used, the desired effect, or more precisely the dose-response, individualized to the specific patient. The possibility of giving drugs with psychic activity "to effect" in an individual patient is an enormous advantage. We have recently used the approach in children aged 5-10 years with fentanyl (5 mg) lollipops. The children (sitting in their mother's lap) eagerly take the lollipops, place them in their mouths and gradually become heavily "premedicated". When the desired effect is achieved, the lollipop is removed, the child picked up by the anesthesiologist and taken to the operating room. While the child may stir he usually simply opens his eyes, for a few minutes, and then when placed on the operating table returns to "sleep". Respiration is only minimally effected, if at all, and the children readily tolerate a face mask. Adults can be handled in the same fashion, although the dose required is obviously higher. Similar effects can be achieved with topical application of highly concentrated and potent opioids to the nasal mucosa.[24] In a similar fashion, carfentanil and other highly potent opioids can be applied to the skin of animals with bandaids and result in anesthesia in 15-20 minutes (Port JD, unpublished data).

The fact that numerous compounds, with a variety of actions on central nervous system neurotransmitter function, may be applied transmucosally or transdermally is exciting for the potential applications are far beyond that of anesthesiology. Consider for example, that patients may no longer need to purchase and swallow pills but rather apply dermal patches. Similar responses should be possible in patients with acute or chronic pain. Furthermore, all this should be possible, practical, simple (requires no expensive machines), painless (requires no needles) and more controllable than possible at the present time. Consider that patients with chronic, longstanding pain might be able to have continuous pain relief with a patch or a bandaid on his or her skin. Consider that postoperative pain could be handled in the same way. These developments are occurring today and, at least in this authors opinion, have implications beyond our specialty, indeed, beyond the boundaries of what we call, and know as, medicine.

References

1. Knigge KM, Joseph SA: Anatomy of the opioid-systems of the brain.
    Can J Neurol Sci 11:14-23, 1984

2. Knigge KM, Joseph SA, Norton J: Topography of the ACTH-immuno-
    reactive neurons in the basal hypothalamus of the rat brain.
    Brain Res 216:333-341, 1981

3. Pasternak GW: Opiate, enkephalin and endorphin analgesia: Re-
    lations to a single subpopulation of opiate receptors. Neurol
    Oct;31(10):1311-1315, 1981

4. Chen G, Ensoi CR, Bohner B: Drug effects on the disposition of
    active biogenic amines in the CNS. Life Sci 7:1063-1974, 1968

5. Haigler HJ, Adhojanian GK: Serotonin receptors in the brain.
    Fed Proc 36:2159-2164, 1977

6. Moore RY, Bloom FE: Central catecholamine neuron systems:
    Anatomy and physiology. Ann Rev Neurosci 1:129-169, 1978

7. Bartholini G, Pletocher A: Cerebral accumulation and metabolism
    of C14-Copa after selective inhibition of peripheral decarboxy-
    lose. J Pharmacol Exp Ther 161:14-20, 1968

8. Haveman U, Turski L, Schwaz M, Kuschinsky K: On the role of
    GABA-ergic mechanisms in striatum and substantia nigra in
    mediating muscular rigidity. Naunyn-Schmiedeberg's Arch Pharmac
    322(suppl):373, 1983

9. Haveman U, Kuschinsky K: Neurochemical aspects of the opioid
    induced "catatonia". Neurochem Inter 4:199-215, 1982

10. Snyder SH, Goodman RR: Multiple neurotransmitter receptors.
    J Neurochem 35:5-15, 1981

11. Hahn EF, Pasternak GW: Stereochemistry of opiates and their
    receptors. In: Handbook of stereoisonomers. Smith D (ed).
    Boca Ration, CRC Press, 1983

12. Kuhan MJ, Pasternak GW: Analgesics: Neurochemical, behavioral
    and clinical perspectives. New York, Raven Press, 1984

13. Leysen JE, Tollenoere JP, Koch MHJ, Laudran P: Differentiation
    of opiate and neurolept receptor binding in rat brain. Eur J
    Pharmacol 43:253-267, 1977

14. De Castro J, Van de Water A, Wouters L, Xhonneux R, Reneman R, Kay B: Comparative study of cardiovascular neurological and metabolic side effects of eight narcotics in dogs. Acta Anaesthesiology Belg 30:5-99, 1979

15. Niemegeers CJE, Schellekens KHL, Van Bever WFM, Janssen PAJ: Sufentanil a very potent and extremely safe intravenous morphine-like compound in mice, rats and dogs. Drug Res 26:1551-1556, 1976

16. Leysen JE, Laduron PM: Receptor binding properties in vitro and in vivo of some long-acting opiates. Arch Int Pharmacodyn Ther 232:343-346, 1978

17. Van Bever WFM, Niemegeers CJE, Schellekens KHL, Janssen PAJ: N-4 substituted 1 (2-arylethyl)-4-piperidinyl-N-phenylproanamides, a novel series of extremely potent analgesics with unusually high safety margin. Drug Res 26:1548-1551, 1976

18. Bovil J, Sebel P, Stanley TH: Opioid analgesics in anesthesia: With particular reference to their use in cardiovascular anesthesia. Anesthesiology (In Press)

19. Verschraegen R, Rosseel MT, Bogaert M, Roly G: Maptazind. In: Use in postoperative pain. Acta Anaesthiol Belg 27(suppl):123-132, 1976

20. Pasternak GW, Childres SR, Snyder SH: Naloxazone, a long-acting opiate antagonist: Effects of analgesia in intact animals and opiate receptor binding in vitro. J Pharmacol Exp Ther 214:455-462, 1980

21. Martin W: Multiple opioid receptors. Life Sci 28:1547-1554, 1981

22. Pasternak GW, Childers SR, Snyder SH: Opiate analgesia: Evidence for mediation by a subpopulation of opiate receptors. Science May 2;208(4443):514-516, 1980

23. Wood PL, Richard JW, Thakur M: Mu opiate isoreceptors: Differentiation with kappa agonists. Life Sci 31:2313-2317, 1982

24. Port J, Stanley TH, Steffey EM: Narcotic inhalation anesthesia. Anesthesiology 57:A344, 1982

25. Port JD, Stanley TH, McJames S: Topical narcotic anesthesia. Anesthesiology 59:A325, 1983

ALFENTANIL

CARL E. ROSOW, M.D., Ph.D.

Alfentanil is a new tetrazole derivative of fentanyl which appears pharmacodynamically similar to the parent drug but which has a more rapid onset and shorter duration of action. It is being tested as an anesthetic supplement, an induction agent, and a postoperative analgesic.

Since the drug is a typical agonist, it will produce the entire spectrum of opioid depressant and stimulant effects. Like fentanyl, alfentanil can produce truncal rigidity after rapid intravenous administration. All of the acute effects are readily reversed by naloxone.[3] In most cases the duration of naloxone should be greater than that of alfentanil. This drug produces morphine-like subjective effects, tolerance, and physical dependence, and it will therefore be subject to narcotic controls.

The primary advantages of this new agent are pharmacokinetic[2,16] (Table 1): (1) Alfentanil and fentanyl are rapidly redistributed after intravenous administration. (2) Both are rapidly metabolized in the liver so the rate of elimination is determined by return of the drug from peripheral tissues to bloodstream. The hepatic extraction ratio of alfentanil is somewhat less than that of fentanyl. (3) Alfentanil is less lipophilic than fentanyl so its volume of distribution is smaller, and less drug is sequestered peripherally. Despite the fact that alfentanil is more highly protein bound and has a lower clearance than fentanyl, the relatively large amount of drug in the plasma causes it to be eliminated much more rapidly. (4) Unlike fentanyl, alfentanil is predominantly unionized in plasma. This large proportion of diffusible drug may explain why the peak effect occurs in only 60 - 90 seconds after i.v. administration.

Table 1. Comparative pharmacokinetics of fentanyl and alfentanil in
          humans.*

	FENTANYL	ALFENTANIL
$T_{\frac{1}{2}}$ elimination (hr)	3.7	1.6
Volume distribution (L/kg)	4.2	0.86
Protein bound fraction (%)	84	92
Clearance (ml/kg/min)	11.6	6.4
Lipid solubility (octanol:water)	860:1	130:1
pK_a	8.4	6.5
Unionized fraction at pH 7.4 (%)	9	89
Hepatic extraction	0.62	0.49

* Modified from Stanski and Hug[16]

Alfentanil has roughly one-third the peak analgesic potency and
one-third the duration of fentanyl.[7] Doses of 10 - 20 μg/kg produce
intense analgesia and respiratory depression for only 15 - 20
minutes.[13,14] In animals,[4] and probably in humans, alfentanil shows less
tendency than fentanyl to cumulate after repeated doses. Sedation,
cerebrovascular effects, and EEG changes are similar to those seen with
fentanyl.[8,11] The cardiovascular effects appear to be small,[5,15] although
rapid administration may produce hypotension.[1] The frequency of nausea
and vomiting is high for both alfentanil and fentanyl in ambulatory
surgical patients.[13]

Most of the clinical studies on alfentanil have investigated its
intraoperative use, particularly in short procedures. Compared to
fentanyl, it can be used to produce a more intense analgesic effect
without prolonging recovery time. The drug is easily given by
intermittent bolus injections, but in longer procedures continuous
infusion may be more convenient.[10] Alfentanil has been used with both
bolus and infusion techniques to produce sleep and analgesia for cardiac
surgery.[5] Patients have tolerated total doses as high as 2,250 μg/kg for
these long procedures.

Stanski and Hug[16] and others have suggested that plasma levels of
200 - 500 ng/ml are probably sufficient for surgical analgesia, and
spontaneous ventilation may return at levels of 100 - 200 ng/ml. It
should be noted that there is still substantial disagreement in the

literature on the specific values for alfentanil's half-life, clearance, and volume of distribution. Better agreement will be necessary before clinically reliable guidelines can be calculated for drug infusions. Titrating to an analgesic endpoint in the awake patient, however, appears to be relatively easy. Alfentanil has been shown to be suitable for the treatment of postoperative pain using a demand analgesia apparatus.[6]

High doses (100 - 200 µg/kg) without hypnotics can produce an anesthetic state in 1 to 2 minutes.[9,12] Coadministration of a muscle relaxant is mandatory, since rigidity will also be rapid in onset. Patients can usually be extubated in 1 to 2 hours without naloxone reversal. The need for postoperative analgesics may be greatly reduced in these patients, and care must be taken if supplemental analgesics or sedatives are given during the immediate postoperative period.

In summary, alfentanil is pharmacologically quite similar to fentanyl but allows greater moment-to-moment control over the intensity of analgesic effect.

REFERENCES

1. Bartkowski RR, McDonnell TE: Alfentanil as an induction agent -- A comparison with thiopental-lidocaine. Anesth Analg 63: 330-334, 1984.
2. Bovill JG, Sebel PS, Blackburn CL, Heykants J: The pharmacokinetics of alfentanil (R 39209): A new opioid analgesic. Anesthesiology 57: 439-443, 1982.
3. Brown JH, Pleuvry BJ: Antagonism of the respiratory effects of alfentanil and fentanyl by naloxone in the conscious rabbit. Br J Anaesth 53: 1033-1037, 1981.
4. Brown JH, Pleuvry BJ, Kay B: Respiratory effects of a new opiate analgesic, R 39209, in the rabbit: Comparison with fentanyl. Br J Anaesth 52: 1101-1106, 1980.
5. De Lange S, Stanley TH, Boscoe MJ: Alfentanil-oxygen anaesthesia for coronary artery surgery. Br J Anaesth 53: 1291-1296, 1981.
6. Kay B: Use of an on-demand analgesia computer (ODAC) and a comparison of the rate of use of fentanyl and alfentanyl. Anaesthesia 36: 949-951, 1981.
7. Kay B, Pleuvry B: Human volunteer studies of alfentanyl (R 39209), a new short-acting narcotic analgesic. Anaesthesia 35: 952-956, 1980.
8. Levy WJ, McDonnell TE: EEG changes with alfentanil anesthesia [Abstract]. Anesthesiology 57(3A): A-353, 1982.
9. McDonnell TE, Bartkowski RR, Williams JJ: ED_{50} of alfentanil for induction of anesthesia in unpremedicated young adults [Abstract]. Anesthesiology 57(3A): A-352, 1982.

10. McLeskey CH: Alfentanil -- loading dose/continuous infusion for surgical anesthesia [Abstract]. Anesthesiology 57(3A): A-68, 1982.
11. McPherson RW, Johnson RM, Traystman RJ: The effects of alfentanil on the cerebral vasculature [Abstract]. Anesthesiology 57(3A): A-354, 1982.
12. Nauta J, de Lange S, Koopman D, Spierdijk J, van Kleef J, Stanley TH: Anesthetic induction with alfentanil: A new short-acting narcotic analgesic. Anesth Analg 61: 267-272, 1982.
13. Rosow CE, Latta WB, Keegan CR, Nozik DL, Murphy AL, Kimball WR, Philbin DM: Alfentanil and fentanyl in short surgical procedures [Abstract]. Anesthesiology 59(3A): A-345, 1983.
14. Scamman FL, Ghoneim MM, Kortilla K: Ventilatory and mental effects of alfentanil and fentanyl [Abstract]. Anesthesiology 57(3A): A-364, 1982.
15. Sebel PS, Bovill JG, van der Haven A: Cardiovascular effects of alfentanil anaesthesia. Br J Anaesth 54: 1185-1190, 1982.
16. Stanski DR, Hug CC Jr: Alfentanil -- a kinetically predictable narcotic analgesic. Anesthesiology 57: 435-438, 1982.

SUFENTANIL

CARL E. ROSOW, M.D., Ph.D.

Sufentanil is a potent thienyl derivative of fentanyl which is intended for intraoperative use, especially as an analgesic anesthetic for major surgical procedures. It has recently been approved for this indication in the United States.

Sufentanil is a pure opioid agonist, and it has almost thirty times more affinity for morphine (mu) receptors than does fentanyl.[9] It is this high affinity which probably accounts for its analgesic potency: in humans, sufentanil has 600 to 700 times the analgesic effect of morphine and 5 to 10 times that of fentanyl. All of the acute effects are readily reversed by naloxone. The drug produces tolerance and physical dependence and will therefore be subject to narcotic controls.

Sufentanil has about twice the lipid solubility as fentanyl and is rapidly and extensively distributed to all body tissues. Like all of the fentanyl analogues, it has a high metabolic clearance, and the hepatic extraction ratio is 0.72 (72% of hepatic blood flow is cleared of drug in one pass). In animals, the drug is N-dealkylated and O-demethylated, and less than 3% appears unchanged in the urine. The volume of distribution is 2.48 L/kg vs. 4 L/kg for fentanyl.[1] This accounts for sufentanil's shorter elimination half-life (148 minutes). Sufentanil has a slightly faster onset of action and a shorter duration of respiratory depression than fentanyl.[8] Like fentanyl, it appears to be short acting in low doses since termination of its effects depends on rapid redistribution. At higher doses of sufentanil significant plasma levels persist during the elimination phase, and the opioid effects disappear much more slowly.

Almost all of the clinical literature on this drug relates to its use in very high doses (10 to 30 µg/kg) to produce both hypnosis and analgesia for major surgery. The potency and specificity of sufentanil turn out to be an advantage in this setting. In preclinical screening, it was found to produce less cardiovascular toxicity than any known opioid. The therapeutic index (LD_{50}/ED_{50} for analgesia) in ventilated rats was found to be 25,000, while fentanyl and morphine were 277 and 69, respectively.[10] The relevance of these findings to clinical safety remains to be proven, but it is clear that enormous doses of sufentanil are well tolerated in humans. Thirty $\mu g/kg$ of sufentanil is equivalent in analgesic effect to more than 20 mg/kg of morphine, a dose of morphine which would produce substantial morbidity.

The cardiovascular effects of sufentanil have been studied extensively and appear to be the same as those of fentanyl.[5,7] There is no histamine release,[6] mild to moderate vasodilation, and bradycardia. After high doses of sufentanil or fentanyl the hemodynamic and hormonal responses to surgery are greatly attenuated, although some responses may still occur.[4] Sufentanil can also produce dose-related sedation progressing to hypnosis. These effects are accompanied by increases in delta wave activity on the EEG, a finding common to most opioids.[2] Rapid administration of sufentanil can produce the syndrome of chest wall rigidity seen after fentanyl. Of course, very high doses will produce prolonged respiratory depression, so facilities for postoperative ventilation must be available.

Studies are now being done using lower doses of sufentanil for conventional balanced anesthesia. There have been no reports of untoward effects or adverse interactions with commonly used anesthetic agents. The use of sufentanil as an analgesic in awake patients has only been reported in one open trial,[3] but there is no reason to doubt that it could be given safely and efficaciously. Of course, the formulation being used currently is inappropriate for this indication: each ml contains 50 μg of sufentanil citrate, which is equivalent to nearly 50 mg of morphine.

The combination of high lipid solubility and high affinity for opiate receptors makes this opioid an attractive choice for epidural administration. It should produce a highly segmental pattern of analgesia with a much more rapid onset and shorter duration than that of morphine. Tests of epidural sufentanil are currently underway.

In summary, sufentanil is a potent analgesic which seems to be at least as good as fentanyl in its ability to produce hypnosis and stable hemodynamic conditions during surgery and is somewhat shorter-acting.

REFERENCES

1. Bovill JG, Sebel PS, Blackburn CL, Heykants J: Kinetics of alfentanil and sufentanil: A comparison [Abstract]. Anesthesiology 55(3A): A-174, 1981.
2. Bovill JG, Sebel PS, Wauquier A, Rog P: Electroenchephalographic effects of sufentanil anesthesia in man. Br J Anaesth 54: 45-52, 1982.
3. Cathelin M, Viguer R, Malki A, Viars P: Le citrate de sufentanil administré par voie intra-musculaire. Activité analgésique chez l'homme conscient. Anesth Analg [Paris] 38: 21-25, 1981.
4. De Lange S, Boscoe MJ, Stanley TH, de Bruijn N, Philbin DM, Coggins CH: ADH and growth hormone responses during coronary artery surgery with sufentanil-O_2 and alfentanil-O_2 anesthesia in man. Anesth Analg 61: 434-438, 1982.
5. Larsen R, Sonntag H, Schenk H-D, Radke J, Hilfiker O: Die Wirkungen von Sufentanil und Fentanyl auf Hämodynamik, Coronardurchbluting und myocardialen Metabolismus des Menschen. Anaesthesist 29: 277-279, 1980.
6. Rosow CE, Philbin DM, Keegan CR, Moss J: Hemodynamics and histamine release during induction with sufentanil or fentanyl. Anesthesiology 60: 489-491, 1984.
7. Sebel PS, Bovill JG: Cardiovascular effects of sufentanil anesthesia: A study in patients undergoing cardiac surgery. Anesth Analg 61: 115-119, 1982.
8. Smith NT, Dec-Silver H, Harrison WK, Sanford TJ, Gillig J: A comparison among morphine, fentanyl and sufentanil anesthesia for open-heart surgery: Induction, emergence and extubation [Abstract]. Anesthesiology 57(3A): A-291, 1982.
9. Stahl KD, van Bever W, Janssen P, Simon EJ: Receptor affinity and pharmacological potency of a series of narcotic analgesic, anti-diarrheal and neuroleptic drugs. Eur J Pharmacol 46: 199-205, 1977.
10. Van Bever WFM, Niemegeers CJE, Schellekens KHL, Janssen PAJ: N-4-substituted 1-(2-arylethyl)-4-piperidinyl-N-phenylpropanamides, a novel series of extremely potent analgesics with unusually high safety margin. Arzneimittelforsch 26: 1548-1551, 1976.

AGONIST-ANTAGONISTS AND THEIR RECEPTORS

CARL E. ROSOW, M.D., Ph.D.

1. GENERAL PROPERTIES

Although nalorphine (N-allylnormorphine, the prototype agonist-antagonist) was known to be an antagonist in the 1920s, its analgesic properties were not discovered until 1954.[6,9] The traditional analgesic screens in animals such as the hotplate or tail-flick test had not indicated any analgesic activity for this compound. Lasagna and Beecher[17] discovered serendipitously that nalorphine was equipotent as an analgesic with morphine. Wikler[32] showed that administration of nalorphine to morphine dependent subjects not only failed to produce euphoria, but precipitated withdrawal.

The pharmacologic effects of nalorphine cannot be explained simply as a combination of morphine and antimorphine actions. Increasing the dose of nalorphine beyond 10 mg appears to produce relatively little increase in analgesia or respiratory depression.[15] In Lasagna and Beecher's original study large numbers of the test subjects had severe psychotomimetic reactions. The distressing hallucinations and dysphoria made nalorphine unacceptable for clinical use as an analgesic, but it gave the first indication that potent analgesia and addiction liability might be separated.

We now know that members of this class of drugs can be very potent analgesics which share most of morphine's side effects. In other ways they differ substantially from the agonists. These differences may or may not prove to be clinically advantageous, but they have been invaluable in furthering our knowledge of opiate action, pain, and addiction. The interested reader is referred to the excellent reviews by Houde[9] and Braude et al..[3]

2. RECEPTOR MECHANISMS

In 1967 Martin postulated his theory of receptor dualism to explain these unique pharmacologic properties. In brief, he described two receptors: one for morphine-like drugs and one for nalorphine-like drugs. According to this According to this model, morphine and nalorphine produce their agonist effects by interactions with separate receptors. Nalorphine has affinity for morphine receptors as well, but it lacks efficacy at these sites and therefore competitively antagonizes morphine. Naloxone has affinity for both receptors and efficacy at neither. Since nalorphine has limited ability to produce many of the opioid effects, it is frequently described as a partial agonist.

Martin has since expanded his theory to incorporate three types of opioid receptors, each one mediating different effects (Table 1).[18,19]

Table 1. Opiate receptor subtypes.*

TEST SYSTEM	RECEPTOR		
	Mu	Kappa	Sigma
Analgesia	Yes	Yes	No
Respiration	Depression	Depression	Stimulation
Behavior	Euphoria	Sedation	Dysphoria
Pupil	Miosis	Miosis	Mydriasis
Morphine Withdrawal	Suppression	No Suppression	No Suppression

* [Modified from Martin et al.[19]]

An opioid may be an agonist, partial agonist, or antagonist at each receptor (Table 2). This hypothetical classification does not fully explain all the data, but it is a useful way to conceptualize much of the clinical pharmacology of these agents. It also gives the correct impression that the opioid agonist-antagonists are a heterogeneous group of drugs.

Broadly speaking, the agonist-antagonists may be grouped into those acting at mu receptors and those acting at kappa receptors. Partial agonists at the mu receptor (e.g., buprenorphine) have high affinity but limited efficacy at morphine receptors. They produce morphine-like

Table 2. Hypothetical receptor interactions for various opioids.[*]

DRUG	RECEPTOR		
	Mu	Kappa	Sigma
Morphine	Agonist	Agonist	0
Buprenorphine	P. Agon.	0	0
Profadol	P. Agon.	0	0
Propiram	P. Agon.	0	0
Dezocine	P. Agon.	0	0
Meptazinol	P. Agon. [†]	0	0
Nalorphine	Antag	P. Agon.	Agon.
Pentazocine	Antag.	P. Agon.	Agon.
Butorphanol	Antag. [§]	P. Agon.	Agon.
Nalbuphine	Antag.[**]	P. Agon.	Agon.
Naloxone	Antag.	Antag.	Antag.

[*] Abbreviations: Agon. = Agonist; P. Agon. = Partial Agonist;
      Antag. = Antagonist; 0 = No Activity
[†] Other mechanisms appeared to be involved in the analgesic effect
   as well.
[§] An opioid antagonist in animals but does not precipitate
   abstinence in humans.
[**] May also have partial agonistic activity.

effects but have shallow dose-response curves. Because they bind so
strongly they may displace pure agonists and therefore act as morphine
antagonists. None of these drugs are currently approved for use in the
United States. The kappa type agonist-antagonists (e.g., nalorphine) act
as competitive antagonists at the mu receptor, but produce their analgesic
effects by agonist activity at kappa receptors. Pentazocine, nalbupine,
and butorphanol belong to this class. The dysphoria or hallucinations
occasionally produced by members of this class are thought to be mediated
by a third type of receptor, called sigma. It is not clear at this time
whether one group of drugs will prove to be clinically superior. Neither
agonist vs. antagonist potency (Table 3) nor putative receptor
interactions have turned out to be good predictors for patient acceptance
or abuse liability.[10]

Table 3. Agonist/antagonist potency in humans.

DRUG	ANALGESIC POTENCY	MORPHINE ANTAGONIST POTENCY
Morphine	1	0
Buprenorphine	25	10
Butorphanol	5	NA *
Nalorphine	1	1
Nalbuphine	1	0.25
Pentazocine	0.25	0.02
Propiram	0.09	0.005

* Similar to nalbuphine in animals, antagonism not demonstrated in humans.

3. SPECIFIC DRUGS

Pentazocine

Pentazocine is presumed to be an agonist at kappa and sigma receptors and a weak antagonist at mu receptors (vide supra). It was the first opioid antagonist marketed for its analgesic properties.[4] It is effective orally and parenterally (oral:parenteral = 4:1). Although it is well absorbed, there is more than 80% first-pass metabolism. Blood levels increase rapidly, and peak effects occur 15 – 60 minutes after intramuscular injection.

Pentazocine is primarily metabolized by oxidation and glucuronide conjugation in the liver, and a small amount appears unchanged in the urine. The elimination half-life is between 2 and 3 hours, but clinically pentazocine is shorter acting than morphine.

Intramuscular doses of 30 to 50 mg produce analgesia, sedation, and respiratory depression roughly equivalent to 10 mg morphine. In contrast to morphine or meperidine, pentazocine has a very limited ability to lower the minimum alveolar concentration (MAC) for cyclopropane in dogs.[8] This has been interpreted by some as an indication of limited analgesic efficacy.

Much has been made of the so-called "ceiling effect" for the respiratory depressant effects of agonist-antagonists, but overdosage of pentazocine may still produce marked depression of ventilation. Respiratory depression may be reversed with naloxone but not nalorphine.

Pentazocine is a very weak antagonist (roughly 1/50 as potent as nalorphine), so it is not clinically useful for reversal of morphine. In physically dependent subjects and in patients regularly taking opioid agonists, pentazocine may precipitate withdrawal.

The side effects are similar in most respects to morphine. Pentazocine has less tendency than morphine to produce constipation and increases in biliary pressure, and this may be useful under certain circumstances.[26]

The hemodynamic effects deserve special mention. In contrast, to the agonists, pentazocine can increase heart rate, systemic and pulmonary arterial pressure, and increase cardiac work.[1] These changes are accompanied by increases in plasma catecholamines and are apparently not due to hypercarbia.[31] Myocardial oxygen consumption probably increases (although this has not been measured), so pentazocine is generally thought to be a poor choice for use in myocardial ischemia or infarct.

The main limitation to the usefulness of this drug is its tendency to produce dysphoria, bad dreams, or outright hallucinations (usually visual). The frequency has been reported as anywhere from 3 to 33%. These effects are reversible by naloxone.

It is now clear that therapeutic doses of pentazocine can produce morphine-like euphoria in addicts, and the drug does have more abuse potential than originally thought. Nevertheless, the illicit use of pentazocine is less than that of codeine or propoxyphene and much less than morphine or meperidine.

Butorphanol

Butorphanol is thought to be a kappa and sigma agonist, but its interaction with mu receptors is not as clear. Despite the fact that it antagonizes morphine in animals, it neither precipitates nor suppresses withdrawal in human subjects dependent on high doses of morphine.[11,13]

The time effect curve for analgesia after intramuscular injection is very similar to morphine. The half-life for elimination in humans is 2.7 hours, while that for morphine is about 3 hours.[24] Butorphanol undergoes extensive hepatic biotransformation (primarily N-dealkylation, glucuronidation, and O-hydroxylation), and less than 5% is excreted unchanged in the urine.

The analgesic potency of butorphanol is about five times that of morphine. In postsurgical patients intramuscular administration of 2 mg produces analgesia and respiratory depression similar to 10 mg morphine. There is probably a ceiling effect for respiratory depression, since 2 or 4 mg of butorphanol produce similar displacement of the CO_2 response curve.[14,23] There is some evidence that butorphanol has a ceiling effect for analgesia as well. In dogs, butorphanol produces only limited decreases in enflurane MAC.[22] Clinical data show that even very large doses (0.3–1.0 mg/kg i.v.) do not induce a state of "anesthesia" as might be seen with morphine.[30] On the other hand, butorphanol suppresses the autonomic responses to endotracheal intubation in a dose-related manner over a range of 0.025 to 0.10 mg/kg i.v.[29]

Butorphanol can fairly reliably produce in man what Martin et al.[19] have described in animals as a state of "apathetic sedation." This may cause some confusion for the nursing staff, since sedation is frequently disproportionate to the observed level of respiratory depression or the patient's subjective reports of pain. Whether or not this sedation is useful will depend upon the clinical situation. Butorphanol can also produce dysphoric reactions like pentazocine, but the incidence is much lower. Visual hallucinations occurred in only 0.1% of the 1,500 patients studied during Phase III testing.[5] It is possible that unpleasant mental effects occur more frequently in patients who have been treated chronically with opioid agonists.

Butorphanol produces about one-half the incidence of nausea and vomiting when compared with morphine in a postoperative setting. Like pentazocine, it produces much less increase in intrabiliary pressure.[27] The hemodynamic effects are reminiscent of pentazocine's. Butorphanol can elevate pulmonary artery pressure, although heart rate and systemic pressure usually decrease slightly.[25] Until these effects are documented more thoroughly butorphanol should be used cautiously in patients with myocardial insufficiency or ischemia.

Thus far, butorphanol has not been subject to a large amount of diversion or elicit use. Whether it will have less abuse liability than pentazocine remains to be seen.

Nalbuphine

Like pentazocine and butorphanol nalbuphine is apparently a kappa and sigma agonist. Unlike either of these drugs it is a moderately potent mu antagonist (approximately one-fourth as potent as nalorphine). In subjects dependent upon 60 mg of morphine per day nalbuphine caused dose-related precipitated abstinence.[12] The agonist effects of nalbuphine can be antagonized with naloxone, but not nalorphine.

After intramuscular injection of 10 mg, peak plasma concentration occurs at 30 minutes, and the elimination half-life is 5.1 hours. The peak analgesic effect occurs at 45 - 60 minutes and lasts slightly longer than morphine. The human metabolic pathways for nalbuphine have not been completely determined, but only small amounts are excreted unchanged in the urine.

As an analgesic and respiratory depressant intramuscular nalbuphine is approximately equipotent with morphine (0.8 to 1.1 times morphine in terms of total analgesia) in studies of postoperative pain.[2,21] Reasonable doses for acute pain in non-tolerant individuals would therefore be 10 to 20 mg, i.m. or s.c.

Both respiratory depression and analgesia appear to be limited with this agent. Respiratory depression reaches a maximum after 30 mg/70 kg and does not increase. The amount of respiratory depression produced by this dose is equal intensity to that from 20 mg/70 kg of morphine. Gal et al.[7] measured respiratory depression and analgesia in volunteers given intravenous nalbuphine. They found that CO_2 responses and reduction of experimentally-induced ischemic pain were maximal after 0.15 mg/kg of the drug. No such plateau effects were found when morphine was studied. Murphy and Hug[22] found that nalbuphine has a very limited ability to lower enflurane MAC in dogs. Lake et al.[16] showed that even doses of nalbuphine as high as 2 - 3 mg/kg do not reliably produce hypnosis or attenuate responses to painful stimuli in patients undergoing coronary artery or mitral valve surgery. These data and the information already presented on butorphanol indicate that these drugs are partial analgesic agonists. One would predict they would be poor choices in situations where extremely high doses of analgesics are used to produce complete anesthesia (e.g., cardiac surgery).

The primary side effect of nalbuphine is sedation which is similar in type and incidence to that produced by butorphanol. Dysphoria and

90

psychotomimetic reactions can occur, but the reported incidence is much lower than with pentazocine.

Unlike pentazocine or butorphanol, nalbuphine does not appear to increase pulmonary artery pressure or produce changes which might increase myocardial oxygen demand.[28] The drug is also well tolerated in the setting of acute myocardial infarction.

The smooth muscle effects in the gut, biliary tree, and bladder are less than those of pure agonists.[20]

As stated above, nalbuphine will not maintain a morphine or heroin addiction but will precipitate withdrawal. For this reason, nalbuphine should be used cautiously, if at all, in patients with significant prior exposure to opioid agonists. Based upon limited experience, the abuse liability of nalbuphine is probably similar to pentazocine.

REFERENCES

1. Alderman EL, Barry WH, Graham AF, Harrison DC: Hemodynamic effects of morphine and pentazocine differ in cardiac patients. N Engl J Med 287: 623-627, 1972.
2. Beaver WT, Feise GA: A comparison of the analgesic effect of intramuscular nalbuphine and morphine in patients with postoperative pain. J Pharmacol Exp Ther 204: 487-496, 1978.
3. Braude MC, Harris LS, May EL, Smith JP, Villarreal JE (Eds.): Narcotic Antagonists (Advances in Biochemical Psychopharmacology, Vol. 8). New York, Raven Press, 1973.
4. Brogden RN, Speight TM, Avery GS: Pentazocine: A review of its pharmacological properties, therapeutic efficacy and dependence liability. Drugs 5: 6-91, 1973.
5. Caruso FS, Pircio AW, Madissoo H, Smyth RD, Pachter IJ: Butorphanol, Pharmacological and Biochemical Properties of Drug Substances, Vol. 2. Edited by Goldberg ME. Washington, DC, American Pharmaceutical Association, Academy of Pharmaceutical Sciences, 1979, pp 19-57.
6. Eddy NB, May EL: The search for a better analgesic. Science 181: 407-414, 1973.
7. Gal TJ, Di Fazio CA, Moscicki J: Analgesic and respiratory depressant activity of nalbuphine: A comparison with morphine. Anesthesiology 57: 367-374, 1982.
8. Hoffman JC, Di Fazio CA: The anesthesia-sparing effect of pentazocine, meperidine, and morphine. Arch Int Pharmacodyn Ther 186: 261-268, 1970.
9. Houde RW: Analgesic effectiveness of the narcotic agonist-antagonists. Br J Clin Pharmacol 7: 2975-3085, 1979.
10. Jasinski DR: Human pharmacology of narcotic antagonists. Br J Clin Pharmacol 7: 2875-2905, 1979.

11. Jasinski DR, Griffith JD, Pevnick JS, Clark SC: Progress report on studies from the clinical pharmacology section of the NIDA Addiction Research Center, Problems of Drug Dependence 1975. Proceedings of the 37th Annual Scientific Meeting, Committee on Problems of Drug Dependence. Washington DC, National Academy of Sciences, 1975, pp 121-161.

12. Jasinski DR, Mansky PA: Evaluation of nalbuphine for abuse potential. Clin Pharmacol Ther 13: 78-90, 1972.

13. Jasinski DR, Pevnick JS, Griffith JD, Gorodetzky CW, Cone EJ: Progress report on studies from the clinical pharmacology section of the NIDA Addiction Research Center, Problems of Drug Dependence 1976. Proceedings of the 38th Annual Scientific Meeting, Committee on Problems of Drug Dependence. Washington DC, National Academy of Sciences, 1976, pp 112-148.

14. Kallos T, Caruso FS: Respiratory effects of butorphanol and pethidine. Anaesthesia 34: 633-637, 1979.

15. Keats AS, Telford J: Studies of analgesic drugs. X. Respiratory effects of narcotic antagonists. J Pharmacol Exp Ther 151: 126-132, 1966.

16. Lake CL, Duckworth EN, Di Fazio CA, Durbin CG, Magruder MR: Cardiovascular effects of nalbuphine in patients with coronary or valvular heart disease. Anesthesiology 57: 498-503, 1982.

17. Lasagna L, Beecher HK: The analgesic effectiveness of nalorphine and nalorphine-morphine combinations in man.   J Pharmacol Exp Ther 112: 356-363, 1954.

18. Martin WR: History and development of mixed opioid agonists, partial agonists and antagonists. Br J Clin Pharmacol 7: 273S-279S, 1979.

19. Martin WR, Eades CG, Thompson JA, Huppler RE, Gilbert PE: The effects of morphine- and nalorphine-like drugs in the non-dependent and morphine-dependent chronic spinal dog.   J Pharmacol Exp Ther 197: 517-532, 1976.

20. McCammon RL, Stoelting RK, Madura JA: Effects of butorphanol, nalbuphine, and fentanyl on intrabiliary tract dynamics.   Anesth Analg 63: 139-142, 1984.

21. Miller RR: Evaluation of nalbuphine hydrochloride.   Am J Hosp Pharm 37: 942-949, 1980.

22. Murphy MR, Hug CC: The enflurane sparing effect of morphine, butorphanol and nalbuphine. Anesthesiology 57: 489-492, 1982.

23. Nagashima H, Karamanian A, Malovany R, Radnay P, Ang M, Koerner S, Foldes F: Respiratory and circulatory effects of intravenous butorphanol and morphine. Clin Pharmacol Ther 19: 738-745, 1976.

24. Pittman KA, Smyth RD, Mayol RF: Serum levels of butorphanol by radioimmunoassay.   J Pharm Sci 69: 160-163, 1980.

25. Popio KA, Jackson DH, Ross AM, Schreiner BF, Yu PN: Hemodynamic and respiratory effects of morphine and butorphanol.   Clin Pharmacol Ther 23: 281-287, 1978.

26. Radnay PA, Brodman E, Mankikar D, Duncalf D: The effect of equianalgesic doses of fentanyl, morphine, meperidine, and pentazocine on common bile duct pressure. Anaesthesist 29: 26-29, 1980.

27. Radnay PA, Duncalf D, Novakovic M, and Benoit J: Effect of fentanyl, morphine, meperidine, butorphanol and naloxone on common bile duct pressure [Abstract]. Anesthesiology 57(3A): A-351, 1982.

28. Romagnoli A, Keats AS: Comparative hemodynamic effects of nalbuphine and morphine in patients with coronary artery disease. Cardiovasc Dis Bull Texas Heart Inst 5: 19-24, 1978.

29. Rosow CE, Keegan CR: Butorphanol vs. morphine: Dose-related suppression of the response to intubation [Abstract]. Anesth Analg 63: 270, 1984.

30. Stanley TH, Reddy P, Gilmore S, Bennett G: The cardiovascular effects of high-dose butorphanol-nitrous oxide anaesthesia before and during operation. Can Anaesth Soc J 30: 337-341, 1983.

31. Tammisto T, Jaattela A, Nikki P, Takki S: Effect of pentazocine and pethidine on plasma catecholamine levels. Ann Clin Res 3: 22-29, 1971.

32. Wikler A, Fraser HF, Isbell H: N-allylnormorphine: Effects of single doses and precipitation of acute "abstinence syndromes" during addiction to morphine, methadone or heroin in man (post-addicts). J Pharmacol Exp Ther 109: 8-20, 1953.

NEW USES FOR AGONIST-ANTAGONISTS IN ANESTHESIA

Elemer K. Zsigmond, M.D.

The introduction of neuroleptanalgesia by De Castro and Mundeleer opened a new epoch in anesthesiology, since many of the side effects associated with the deep planes of inhalational anesthetics were obviated. The separate and appropriate dosing of droperidol and fentanyl allowed the safe conduct of surgery with minimal adverse endocrine and metabolic sequelae. The introduction of benzodiazepines provided another safe, alternate technique; ataract-analgesia with the combination of diazepam-fentanyl or flunitrazepam-fentanyl has been used during the past two decades. The introduction of the highly specific narcotic antagonist, naloxone, further enhanced the safety of neurolept- or ataract-analgesia, since reversal of the respiratory depression could be carried out with safety.

The introduction of an agonist-antagonist offered another alternative to neuroleptanalgesia: pentazocine-droperidol and pentazocine-diazepam combinations with or without $N_2O:O_2$. In the next decade, butorphanol, nalbuphine and buprenorphine among the multitude of new agonist-antagonists underwent thorough clinical pharmacologic, hemodynamic and endocrine studies. Dr. De Castro discusses his studies on buprenorphine in great detail in this volume, while Dr. Rosow describes the clinical pharmacology and receptors of agonist-antagonists, therefore only the new uses of agonist-antagonists are discussed.

PENTAZOCINE

Analgesic effect. Pentazocine has been used as an analgesic for
postoperative pain, for minor surgical procedures, for relief of painful
diagnostic procedures and for supplementation of inhalational or
regional anesthesia.[1-10]

Balanced anesthesia. Aldrete utilized pentazocine frequently for
awake intubation[11] and laryngoscopy[12] in balanced anesthesia.
Keéri-Szánto and Pomeroy[13] determined the dose requirements: the priming
dose and maintenance dose requirements of pentazocine in combination
with N_2O in urban vs. rural populations and smokers vs. non-smokers.
Although there was a lesser difference between urban vs. rural populations
than between smokers and non-smokers in the primary dose, the maintenance
doses were significantly higher in urban dwellers and smokers than in
their rural and non-smokers counterparts. The accuracy of the graphically
determined mg/kg doses versus time of anesthesia has been validated in
a former publication.[14] There was a linear correlation between the
total dose given and the plasma pentazocine levels found by fluorometric
pentazocine assay. The calculated and observed pentazocine blood levels
correlated well.[13]

The combination of diazepam with pentazocine has been shown to offer
good operative conditions for gynecologic and oral surgery.[15,16,17]
Hatano et al[18] utilized diazepam (0.4 mg/kg) - pentazocine (2.0 mg/kg)
combination for cardiac surgery and observed a moderate depression of
the cardiac output and a moderate increase in peripheral vascular
resistance. Aldrete[19] used a diazepam-pentazocine mixture in a wide
variety of anesthetic applications. He reported excellent amnesia,
moderate analgesia, moderate respiratory depression, lack of histamine
release, no muscle rigidity; but side effects of protracted recovery,

nausea, vomiting and dizziness. De Castro[20] also utilized pentazocine
for analgesic sedation, but observed pre-epileptic EEG patterns after
greater than 200 mg i.v. doses, therefore abandoning it in favor of
buprenorphine. We shared his experience with the limited analgesic
potency of pentazocine as compared to fentanyl, since many patients
undergoing cardiac surgery showed pupillary signs of pain and had
markedly elevated blood pressure and norepinephrine plasma levels during
diazepam-pentazocine-N_2O anesthesia. Indeed, increases in plasma
catecholamines and 17-hydroxycorticosteroid (cortisol) levels were also
observed by Oyama et al[21] in patients anesthetized by pentazocine-$N_2O:O_2$.
These changes may reflect inadequate pain relief, since pain primarily
causes central sympathetic stimulation as reflected in elevated plasma
free norepinephrine concentrations.[22] Because of the dysphoric and
psychotomimetic effects and the addiction liability of pentazocine, the
newer agonist-antagonists replaced it.

BUTORPHANOL

Analgesic effect. Butorphanol has been utilized for pain relief since
double-blind studies established that it is as effective as but safer
than morphine, meperidine and pentazocine for the relief of postoperative
pain. It is 20 times more potent than pentazocine and 5 times more potent
than morphine. Pain relief is present at 30 min and lasts for 4 hours.[23, 31]
When given to 10 volunteers, the respiratory depression as evaluated
to CO_2-response after 4 mg/70 kg butorphanol was equal to that caused
by 10 mg/70 kg morphine.[32] A "ceiling effect" on ventilation was observed
by Nagashima et al.[32] Plasma histamine levels are not increased significantly by butorphanol in dogs[33] and biliary duct pressure increases less
after butorphanol than after i.v. morphine.[34]

Balanced anesthesia. The advantages of butorphanol led to its introduction into intravenous analgesic anesthesia in place of fentanyl by
Dobkin et al.[35] Prior to induction diazepam and atropine or scopolamine was used for premedication.They administered 1.5 to 4.0 mg butorphanol
i.v. prior to a sleep dose of 2-4 mg/kg of thiopental. Pancuronium
was used as muscle relaxant for intubation. Anesthesia was supplemented
with 65% N_2O and additional doses of 0.5-1.0 mg butorphanol. One of
the 53 patients required chlorpromazine to reduce the elevated blood
pressure that remained high despite additional doses. The incidences
of nausea and vomiting were 26% and 13% respectively. In a double-blind
study, Del Pizzo[36] could not differentiate morphine (32.8 mg i.v. total
dose) from butorphanol (6.6 mg i.v. total dose) used for balanced
anesthesia with $N_2O:O_2$. In a double-blind study, no advantage for
butorphanol over fentanyl was found by Zauder.[37] Furthermore, Stehling
and Zauder[37] encountered patients who remained hypertensive despite
additional doses of butorphanol and meperidine in another double-blind
study suggesting that both drugs have a "ceiling effect" for analgesia.
Indeed, recently Stanley et al[38] found that butorphanol even in mega-doses
is unable to block hemodynamic circulatory responses to surgery in
patients undergoing cardiac surgery. The enflurane sparing effect of
butorphanol, nalbuphine, and morphine is limited. In dogs, a "ceiling
effect" was observed by Murphy and Hug[39], for the potentiation of
anesthetics by intravenous anesthetic agents that may explain the limited
capacity of intravenous analgesics to provide complete anesthesia and
blockade of sympathetic autonomic reflexes and circulatory changes instead
of analgesia. This lack of inhibition of sympathetic-responses to autonomic
stimulation during neurolept analgesia or during "pure" analgesic-anesthe-
sia,[40] however, cannot be equated with an analgesic "ceiling", since

these autonomic sympathetic responses cannot be blocked but rather enhanced by even very large doses of analgesic drugs causing per se excessive sympathetic stimulation (De Castro et al).[40] This problem should be further investigated with all the agonist-antagonists.

The marked increase in pulmonary artery pressures by butorphanol observed by Popio et al[41] certainly contraindicates the use of butorphanol in patients in whom such an increase in right ventricular work may be detrimental. Although psychotomimetic effects are less frequent with butorphanol than with morphine, nonetheless they may occur, delaying discharge from the recovery room. Butorphanol has a low physical dependence liability.[42]

Pharmacokinetics. The pharmacokinetics of butorphanol follow a bi-exponential decay curve following a 2 mg/70 kg i.v. injection to normal volunteers. The terminal half-life is 2.7 hours, as determined by a radioimmune-assay. By enzymatic hydrolysis increased amounts of butorphanol in the plasma observed indicates that part of the butorphanol is in its conjugate form. A linear correlation between the injected dose and plasma levels was observed.[43]

NALBUPHINE

Analgesic effect. For perioperative and chronic pain relief, nalbuphine has a well-established place as to effectiveness vs. safety ratio, based on a double-blind controlled study[44] and the Veterans Administration Cooperative Analgesic Study completed in 1970-71.[44-51]

Beaver and Feise[46,47] determined the potency of nalbuphine vs. morphine i.m. for postoperative pain. They found nalbuphine equipotent to morphine or a ratio of 1:1. Oral nalbuphine is about 1/5 as potent as intramuscular nalbuphine.[48] Nalbuphine was also found effective for pain relief in children.[49] Patient acceptance was good and side effects were lower than with morphine. In 153 patients with acute postoperative pain following orthopedic procedures or trauma, Okun found nalbuphine three times as potent as codeine orally in late postoperative pain. In chronic pain of malignancy, nalbuphine proved effective and safe.[51] In all these studies, nalbuphine was found equipotent to morphine. However, in patients who underwent abdominal surgery under enflurane anesthesia in the recovery room for the relief of severe pain, we found that nalbuphine was 2-2.5 times less potent than morphine.*

<u>Circulation</u>. The hemodynamic effects of nalbuphine as compared to morphine were favorable in patients with coronary artery diseases.[52] In 15 patients within 72 hours of acute myocardial infarction both nalbuphine 10 mg and morphine 10 mg were administered intravenously 16 to 24 hours apart in a randomized double-blind manner. Mean intraarterial pressure fell significantly ($p \leqslant 0.05$) after morphine but not after nalbuphine during the one-hour observation period.[53] Both drugs decreased cardiac index, while nalbuphine caused a significant increase in systemic vascular resistance from 1204 to 1379 dsc^{-5} without elevating left ventricular filling pressure. Stroke work index was unchanged after either drug, but the mean velocity of left ventricular fiber shortening was reduced more by nalbuphine than by morphine.[53] Therefore, myocardial work and oxygen requirement had to be reduced proportionately after nalbuphine. This oxygen-sparing effect of nalbuphine over morphine may be beneficial in cardiac patients in need of an analgesic.[53] Lake et al[54] further confirmed this hemodynamic stability following 0.5 to 3.0 mg/kg i.v. injection of nalbuphine in patients with coronary or valvular heart disease.

*Zsigmond, Gronemeyer, Miller and Barabas: Personal communication, 1984.

Ventilatory effects. A "ceiling effect" for respiratory depression by nalbuphine was observed by Romagnoli and Keats;[55] while increasing doses of morphine caused an increased respiratory depression in a linear dose-effect relationship, nalbuphine induced a moderate shift in the CO_2 response curve up to a total dose of 50 mg/70 kg then leveled off. Gal et al[56] confirmed this limited respiratory depression with nalbuphine dose exceeding 0.4 mg/kg total i.v. Utilizing the antagonist effect of nalbuphine, Magruder et al[57] succeeded in reversing narcotic induced respiratory depression by administering 0.1 mg/kg nalbuphine i.v. while the analgesia remained intact. Julien[58] confirmed these findings.

Potentiation of MAC_{50} of inhalational anesthetics. DiFazio and associates[59] showed a potentiation of MAC_{50} of inhalational anesthetic agents that was confirmed by Murphy and Hug[39] with enflurane. The latter authors, however, found a lower potentiation of inhalational anesthetics with nalbuphine or butorphanol than by morphine.

Potentiation of nalbuphine analgesia. An H_1-antagonist, diphenhydramine, was observed to potentiate nalbuphine analgesia in rats by Bluhm, Zsigmond and Winnie.[60] This potentiation was also observed with fentanyl and morphine.

Abuse potential. Nalbuphine has very minimal abuse potential.[61] Therefore it is not a controlled substance and may be stocked in the anesthesia cart or in an emergency medical kit.

Miscellaneous effects. Histamine-liberation with nalbuphine is minimal,* if it ever occurs, and has no clinical importance. It is unlikely to alter vasomotor tone as Muldoon et al[62] demonstrated in canine saphenous vein. Although nalbuphine produced hypothermia at 20°C in mice as Rosow et al showed,[63] these responses were unaffected by raising the temperature to 30°C over a wide range of doses in contrast to other agonists, e.g.

butorphanol, which causes hypothermia at 20°C and an attenuated hypothermic
response at 30°C when given in high doses. Human data on the effect of
nalbuphine on thermoregulation have not been reported as yet.

Balanced anesthesia. Magruder et al[64] and Fahmy[65] found nalbuphine to
possess adequate potency for balanced anesthesia with stable hemodynamics.
Fahmy utilized a double-blind parallel design in 70 patients undergoing
orthopedic surgery. Nalbuphine and morphine, 10 mg/ml were blinded and
randomized. Premedication was study drug 0.1 mg/kg and scopolamine
0.2-0.4 mg 1 hr before anesthesia. Nalbuphine or morphine 0.2-0.4 mg/kg
i.v. was given followed 10 minutes later by diazepam 0.2 mg/kg. Thiopental-
succinylcholine-N_2O-curare sequence was used. 2.0 mg incremental doses
of study drug were then given as needed. Nalbuphine administration caused
no significant changes in arterial and right atrial pressures, heart rate,
stroke volume and ECG, while morphine caused bradycardia and hypotension
in some patients. Adequate analgesia was obtained with either drug.
However, the analgesic potency of nalbuphine was 1.5 to 1.0 as compared
to morphine. Lower incidences of respiratory depression and vomiting
occurred in the nalbuphine than in the morphine group. Camagay and Gomez[66]
confirmed the adequacy of nalbuphine in pediatric patients for balanced
anesthesia with low side-effect liability. No vomiting and no need for
reversal was observed.

In a pilot dose-finding study in 1979 in 47 patients undergoing gynecologic, orthopedic, plastic or abdominal surgery, we found that after
pretreatment with i.v. diazepam and induction with 3-5 mg/kg thiopental,
0.36 $\pm$ 0.18 mg/kg/hr or 25.2 mg/70 kg/hr nalbuphine was required to maintain
adequate analgesia as ascertained by eye-signs, cerebral function and EMG
recordings and hemodynamic data. Anesthesia was supplemented with 66%
N_2O and 0.04 $\pm$ 0.03 mg/kg/hr pancuronium.[67] In 19 patients who underwent

coronary bypass procedures or valvular surgery and in 6 neurosurgical patients whose intracranial pressure was monitored, we determined the hemodynamic effects and dose requirements for maintenance of analgesia. Premedication was hydroxyzine, 2.0 mg/kg i.m. and glycopyrrolate, 3.0 µg/kg i.m. at 6 AM. At 7:30 AM the patients were induced with diazepam 0.4 mg/kg i.v. given over 5 minutes. Eight minutes after completing this injection, we administered pancuronium 0.1 mg/kg i.v. and 2 min later, we gave ketamine 1.0 mg/kg i.v. over 30 seconds. This induction sequence was previously shown to be free of adverse hemodynamic, endocrine and autonomic effects.[68] As soon as intubation was completed, incremental doses of nalbuphine were given until the eye signs, EEG and hemodynamic stability indicated adequate analgesia. We tried to keep the rate pressure-product within $\pm$ 20% range. Hemodynamic measurements showed no significant changes in blood pressure intraarterially recorded, heart rate by ECG, and pulmonary artery pressures measured by Swan Ganz catheter until bypass in the cardiac patients and until skin-closure in the neurosurgical patients. The initial loading dose was 3.0 mg/kg/hr for both groups and was reduced to 0.58 mg/kg/hr for the subsequent intervals. These doses were calculated from the sum of each hourly dose increments as first recommended by Keéri-Szánto.[14]

Cardiothoracic anesthesia. After the pilot studies were completed, we substituted nalbuphine for ketamine as the induction agent. We evaluated the hemodynamic and autonomic effects of ataract-analgesic induction-intubation with:

● diazepam, 0.4 mg/kg/5 min i.v. infusion;

● 10 min waiting period for the development of full effect on CNS;

● nalbuphine, 3.0 mg/kg i.v. infused over 20 minutes;

● pancuronium, 0.1 mg/kg/30 sec i.v.;

- 5 min waiting period;

- intubation without spraying.

For maintenance, nalbuphine 0.5 mg/kg/hr incremental doses i.v. prn in
combination with $N_2O:O_2 = 4: 2$ L/min were used in patients undergoing
coronary-bypass and/or valve replacement. Nalbuphine dosage was based on
pupil size, EEG, or cerebral function monitors and increase in rate pressure
product greater than 20%. There were no significant changes in arterial
blood pressure or heart rate after intubation, surgical incision and
sternotomy, shown in Figures 1 and 2. Pulmonary arterial pressures, which
are good indices of sympathetic stimulation, e.g. inadequate pain relief,
did not increase, as shown in Figure 3.

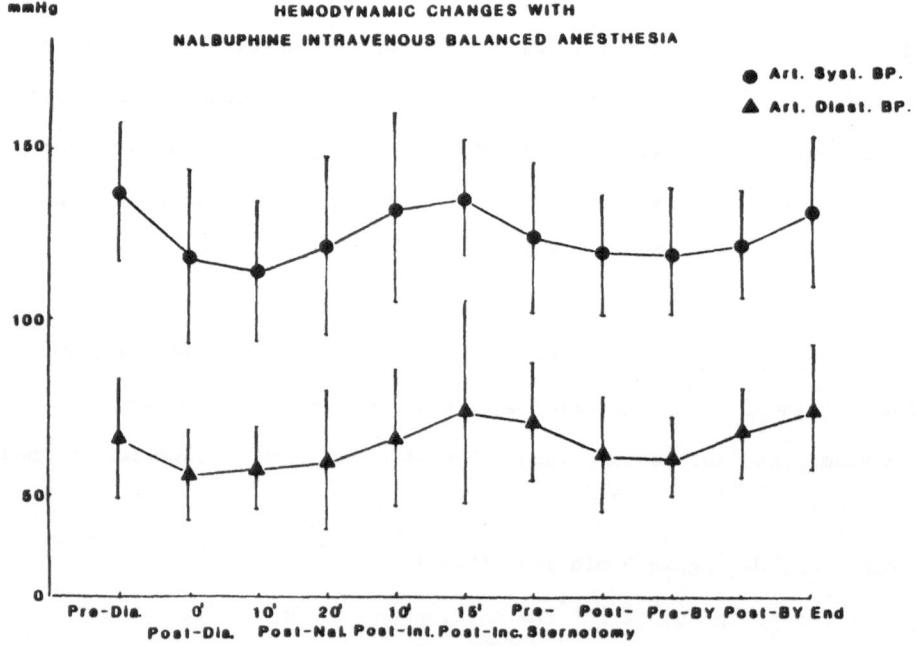

Fig. 1

103

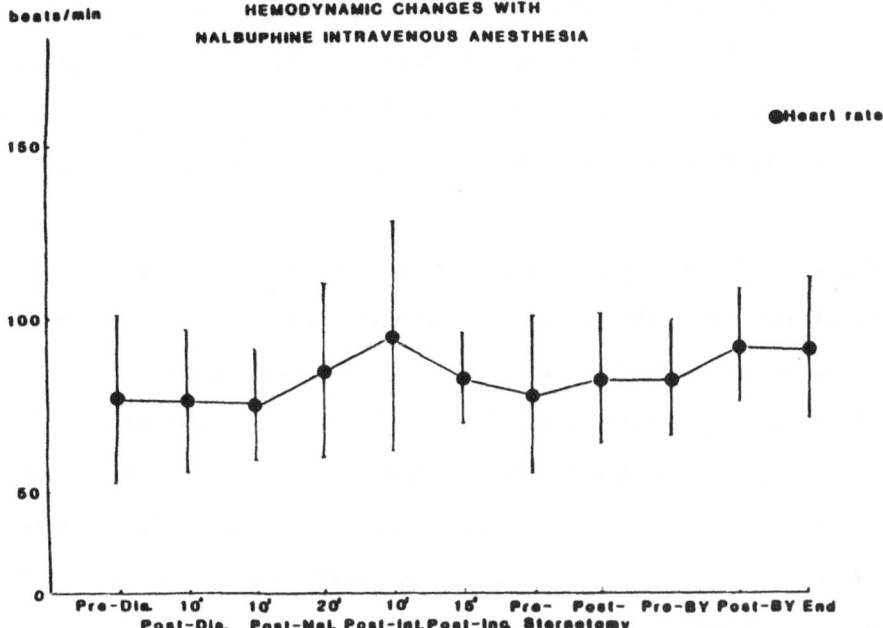

Fig. 2

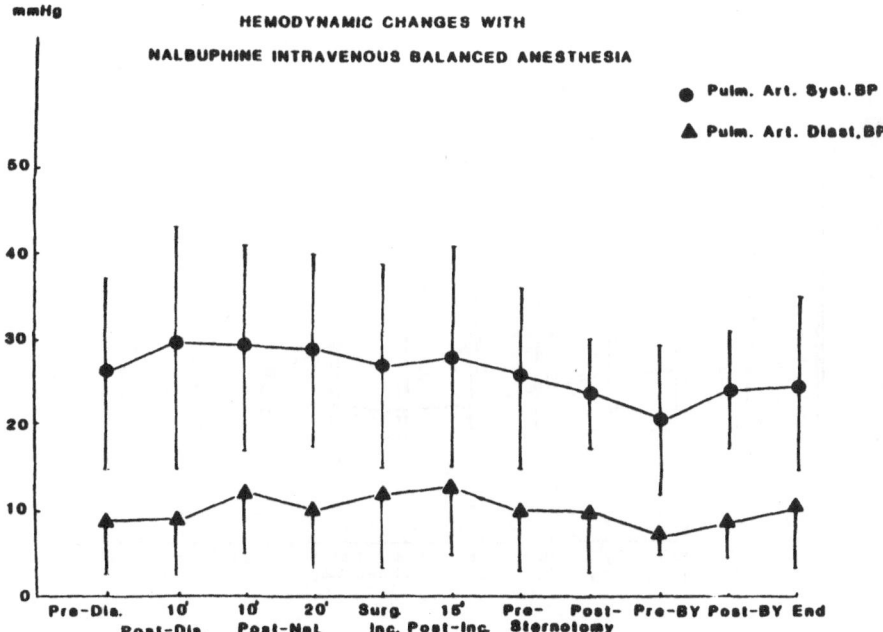

Fig. 3

104

Cardiac index and stroke volume index showed no changes, hence the heart
was not depressed by this technique as shown in Figure 4. Left ventricular
stroke work index was reduced which is beneficial in a cardiac patient.
The most important quality control of an anesthetic technique for both
cardiac surgeons and anesthesiologists, is reflected in the plasma free-
norepinephrine levels. In proof, plasma free norepinephrine levels did not
increase significantly over the levels seen in head-up table-tilt position
at any time during anesthesia and surgery, as shown in Figure 5, indicating
that this technique is effective and safe. Similarly, plasma free
epinephrine and dopamine levels did not change as shown in Figure 5. No
histamine release occurred as shown in Figure 6. Plasma cortisol levels
were significantly elevated after cardiopulmonary bypass as often seen in
this type of procedure as illustrated in Figure 6.

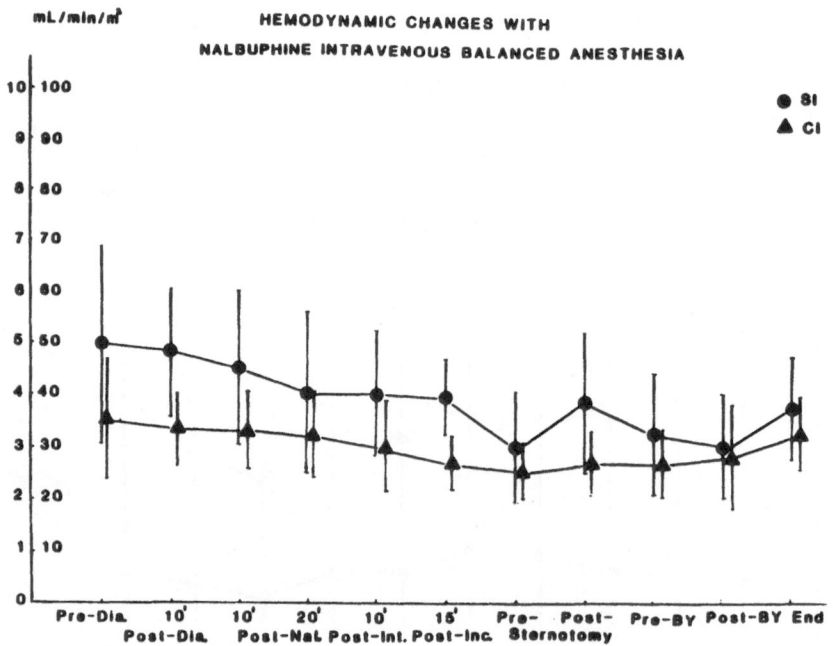

Fig. 4

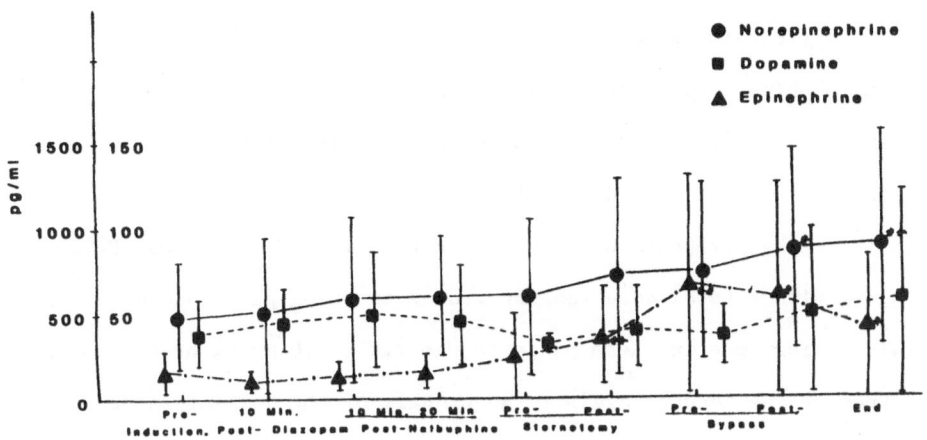

Fig. 5

CHANGES IN CORTISOL AND HISTAMINE LEVELS WITH NALBUPHINE INTRAVENOUS BALANCED ANESTHESIA

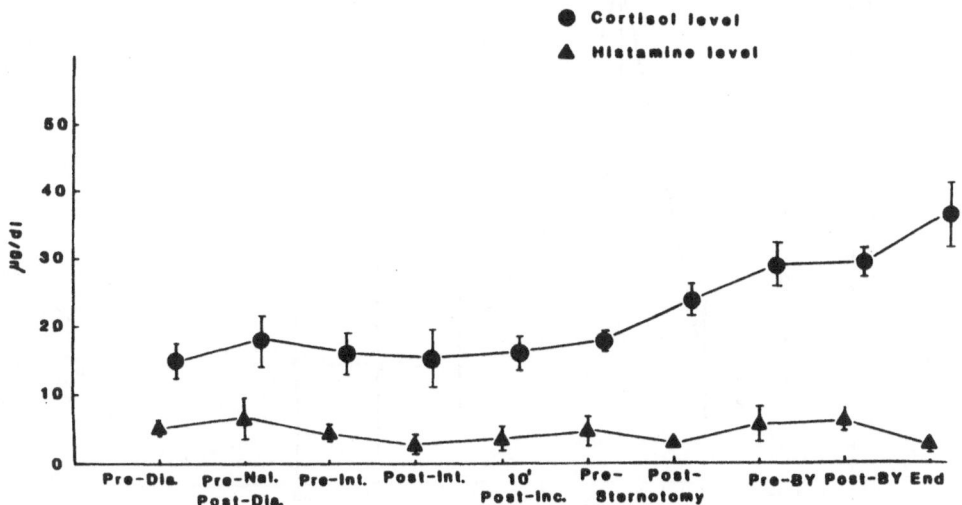

Fig. 6

No chest wall rigidity was observed during infusion of nalbuphine in the spontaneously breathing patients.

The nalbuphine requirements for the total cardiac surgical procedures was fairly high, 18.3 $\pm$ 5.2 mg/kg or a range of 10.0 to 30.0 mg/70 kg per patients. The diazepam requirement was 0.78 $\pm$ 0.18 mg/kg with a range of 0.4 to 1.1 mg/kg per procedure. The pancuronium requirement was 0.25 $\pm$ 0.06 mg/kg with a total dose ranging from 7 to 26 mg per procedure. The initial loading dose in these patients was 7.8 $\pm$ 4.0 mg/kg/hr for the first hour, then it was reduced again to about half of the initial value. Consequently, there was an exponential fall in the dose requirements, almost reaching twice the amount per hour of what is necessary for patients who have already received diazepam-ketamine induction.

Nalbuphine blood level peaked before sternotomy to 7.89 $\pm$ 7.01 µg/ml as shown in Figure 7.

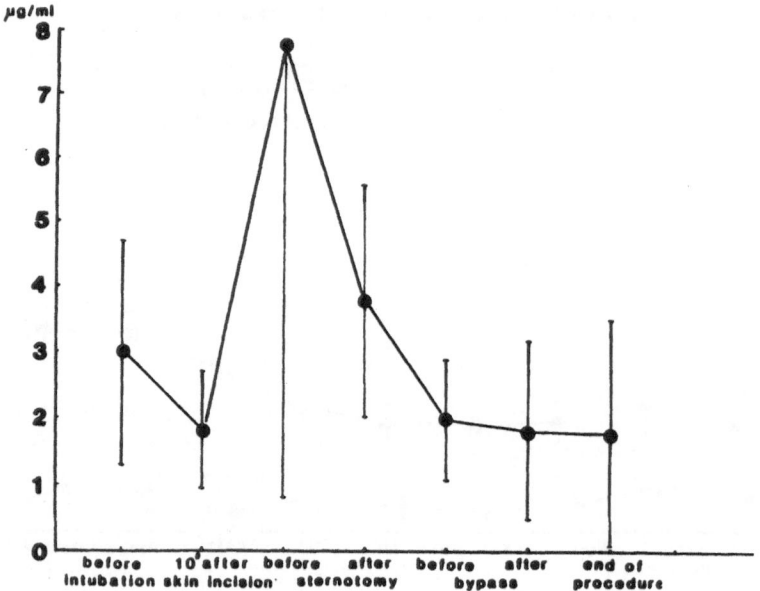

Fig. 7

Afterwards an exponential reduction in blood levels to 1.5 µg/ml was observed as seen in Figure 7.

The advantages of nalbuphine over currently available agents for cardiac anesthesia are: 1) Minimal hemodynamic changes; 2) No histamine release; 3) No chest wall rigidity, allowing the i.v. titration of the loading dose.

<u>Antagonist effect of nalbuphine on the respiratory depression induced by fentanyl.</u> Although Magruder et al[57] demonstrated the reversal of fentanyl-induced respiratory depression by nalbuphine, no hemodynamic measurements nor catecholamine level determinations were made to substantiate the lack of reversal of analgesic effect. We observed in ten patients, that 0.22 ± 0.08 mg/kg nalbuphine completely reversed the respiratory depression without elevation of catecholamines as seen in Figure 8.[69]

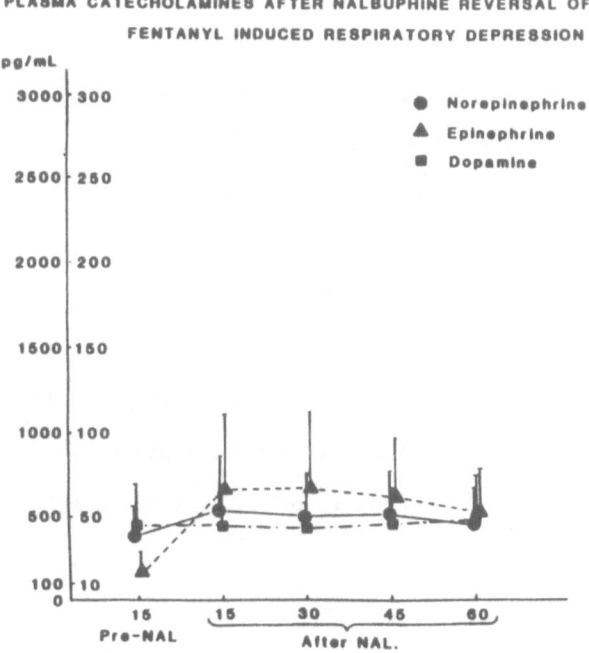

Fig. 8

No significant elevation in systolic blood pressure, pulse rate or Pa_{CO2} occurred at 30, 45 and 60 min following reversal except a significant increase ($p \leqslant 0.05$) at 15 min in systolic pressure that may be explained by the extubation of the patient following reversal. None of the patients had a pain score > 2 units on a 10 unit analogue-scale in the first hour following reversal. Plasma nalbuphine levels ranged from 20-180 ng/ml (measured by HPLC assay) after reversal from 0.1-0.3 mg/kg doses and linearly correlated with the total dose injected.[70] Cortisol levels showed no changes. This is an additional proof that the patient remained pain free. Evidently, nalbuphine is effective for reversal of respiratory depression from narcotic agonists, without reversal of analgesia or adverse circulatory effects.

SUMMARY

Nalbuphine may serve as a safe alternate analgesic agent to fentanyl since it has adequate analgesic potency when used in combination with diazepam and N_2O and assures a stable cardiocirculatory state. Cumulation is low and chest wall rigidity is absent. It causes no histamine release. In lower doses given i.v. it reverses narcotic agonist-induced respiratory depression without reversing analgesia. In higher doses, it supplements thiopental-N_2O or diazepam-ketamine-N_2O anesthesia without adverse hemodynamic or endocrine sequelae. In very high doses, it provides adequate hemodynamic stability and analgesia in combination with diazepam-N_2O for cardiovascular surgery. Because of the lack of histamine-release it may be employed in biliary surgery, in patients with allergic diathesis or in patients with lung disease.

EPILOGUE

At the present and in the near future, diazapam-nalbuphine-N_2O-muscle relaxant anesthesia may replace more hazardous and less reliable anesthetic agents and techniques.

In the distant future, drug research may provide the anesthesiologists with other agonist-antagonists with even greater efficacy and safety. Every effort should be made to achieve this "ideal" analgesic drug.

110

1. Bellville JW, Green J. The respiratory and subjective effects of pentazocine. Clin Pharmacol Therap 6:152, 1965.
2. Bellville JW, Forrest WH, Brown BW. Clinical and statistical methodology for cooperative clinical assays of analgesics. Clin Pharmacol Therap 9:290, 1968.
3. Sadove MS, Balagot RC. Pentazocine: A new nonaddicting analgesic. J Am Med Assoc 193:887, 1965.
4. Tammisto T, Lahdensuu M, Fock G. Pentazocine as a supplement in anesthesia. A clinical comparison of pethidine, fentanyl, and pentazocine in nitrous-oxide-oxygen-relaxant anesthesia. Ann Chir Gynaec Fenn 56:319, 1967.
5. Dundee JW, Clarke RSJ, Loan WB, Hamilton RC. Clinical studies with opiate antagonists. Brit J Anaesth 39: 88, 1967.
6. Alderman EL, Barry WH, Graham AF, Harrison DC. Hemodynamic effects of morphine and pentazocine differ in cardiac patients. New Engl J Med 287:623, 1972.
7. De Castro J, Viars P. Utilisation pratique des analgesiques centraux en anesthesie et reanimation. Ars Medici Sep 23:101, 1968.
8. Dobkin AB, Israel JS, Pislock PA. The metabolic response to pentazocine as a supplement to balanced anaesthesia for major abdominal surgery. Canad Anaesth Soc J 17:485, 1970.
9. Payne JP. The clinical pharmacology of pentazocine. Drugs 5:1, 1973.
10. Ritzow H. Reversability of the fentanyl- and morphine-induced respiratory depression by morphine antagonists. Anaesthetist 22:425, 1973.
11. Aldrete JA, Clapp HW, Fishman J, O'Higgins JW. Pentazepam: A supplementary agent. Anesth Analg 50:498, 1971.
12. Aldrete JA. Respiratory changes during laryngoscopy: Influence of anesthetic technique. ORL Digest 33:29, 1971.
13. Keeri-Szanto M, Pomeroy JR. Atmospheric pollution and pentazocine metabolism. Lancet 1:947, 1971.
14. Keeri-Szanto M. Drug consumption during thiopentone-nitrous oxide-relaxant anesthesia: The preparation and interpretation of time/dose curves. Brit J Anaesth 32:415, 1960.
15. Schoenfeld A, Goldman JA, Levy E. Pentazoncine and diazepam analgesia for minor gynaecological operations. Br J Anaesth 46:385, 1974.
16. Aldrete JA, Tan ST, Carrow DJ, Watts MK. "Pentazepam" (pentazocine-diazepam) supplementing local analgesia for laparascopic sterilization. Anesth Analg 55:177, 1976.
17. Jourde J, Peri G, Menes H et al. The value of associating diazepam and pentazocine in an anesthetic combination in maxillo-facial surgery. Ann Anesthesiol Fr 13:173, 1972.
18. Hatano S, Kean D, Wade MA et al. Diazepam-pentazocine anesthesia for cardiovascular surgery. Canad Anaesth Soc J 21:586, 1974.

19. Aldrete JA. 1980. Somnoanalgesia with Pentazepam. In: Trends in Intravenous Anesthesia. (Eds.) Aldrete JA, Stanley TH. Symposia Specialists, Miami, FL p 433.
20. De Castro J. 1978. les analgésiques centraux et l´anesthésie analgésigue. Elsevier B. Press, S A Bruxelles, Belgium p 97.
21. Oyama T, Takiguchi M, Sato K. Effects of droperidol-pentazocine-N_2O anesthesia on adrenocortical function in man. Canad Anaesth Soc J 18:298, 1971.
22. Kothary SP, Zsigmond EK. Plasma cortisol and norepinephrine after pain relief. Excerp Med ICS 533:1010, 1980.
23. Del Pizzo A. Butorphanol, a new intravenous analgesic: Double-blind compison with morphine sulfate in postoperative patients with moderate or severe pain. Curr Ther Res 20:221, 1976.
24. Tavakoli M, Corssen G, Caruso FS. Butorphanol and morphine. A double-blind comparison of their parenteral analgesic activity. Anesth Analg 55:394, 1976.
25. Dobkin AB, Eamkaow S, Zak S et al. Butorphanol: A double-blind evaluation in postoperative patients with moderate or severe pain. Can Anaesth Soc J 21:600, 1974.
26. Lippmann M, Mok MS, Steen SN et al. Butorphanol and morphine: A double-blind multiple intramuscular dose comparative safety and efficacy study in patients with postoperative pain. Curr Ther Res 21:427, 1977.
27. Dobkin AB, Eamkaow S, Caruso FS. Butorphanol and pentazocine in patients with severe postoperative pain. Clin Pharmacol Therap 18:547, 1975.
28. Dobkin AB, Africa BF, Noveck RJ et al. Butorphanol tartrate: 1. Safety and efficacy in multidose control of postoperative pain. Can Anaesth Soc J 23:596, 1976.
29. Kliman A, Lipson MJ, Warren R et al. Clinical experience with intramuscular butorphanol for the treatment of a variety of chronic pain syndromes. Curr Ther Res 22:105, 1977.
30. Lippmann M, Mok MS, Steen SN et al. Analgesic onset time of intravenous butorphanol in postsurgical patients: A placebo-controlled study. Curr Ther Res 22:276, 1977.
31. Zeedick JF. Efficacy and safety evaluation of butorphanol in postoperative pain. Curr Ther Res 22:707, 1977.
32. Nagashima H, Foldes FF, Karamanian A et al. Respiratory and circulatory effects of intravenous butorphanol and morphine. Clin Pharmacol Therap 19:738, 1976.

112

33. Schurig JE, Cavanagh RL, Buyniski JP. The effects of butorphanol and morphine on pulmonary mechanics, arterial blood pressure and venous plasma histamine levels in anesthetized dogs. Fed Proc 35:546, 1976.
34. Roebel LE, Cavanagh RL, Buyniski JP. Comparative gastrointestinal and biliary tract effects of morphine and butorphanol. J Med 10:225, 1979.
35. Dobkin AB, Arandia HY, Byles PH et al. Butorphanol tartrate. 2. Safety and efficacy in balanced anesthesia. Can Anaesth Soc J 23:601, 1976.
36. DelPizzo A. A double-blind study of the effect of butorphanol compared with morphine in balanced anaesthesia. Can Anaesth Soc J 25:392, 1978.
37. Stehling LC, Zauder HL. Double-blind comparison of butorphanol tartrate and meperidine hydrochloride in balanced anesthesia. J Int Med Res 6:384, 1978.
38. Stanley TH, Reddy P, Gilmore S et al. The cardiovascular effects of high dose butorphanol-nitrous oxide anesthesia before and during operation. Can Anaesth Soc J 30:337, 1983.
39. Murphy MR, Hug CC. The enflurane sparing effect of morphine, butorphanol, and nalbuphine. Anesthesiology 57:489, 1982.
40. De Castro J, Kay B, Reneman A, Van de Water A, Wouters L, Xhonneux R. Comparative study of cardiovascular, neurological and metabolic side effects of eight narcotics in dogs. Acta Anaesth Belg 30:5, 1979.
41. Popio KA, Jackson DH, Ross AM et al. Hemodynamic and respiratory effects of morphine and butorphanol. Clin Pharmacol Therap 23:281, 1978.
42. Jasinski DR, Persnick JS, Griffith JD, Gorodetzky CW, Cove EJ. Progress report on studies from the Clinical Pharmacology Section of the Addiction Research Center, Problems of Drug Dependence, Proceedings, pp 112, 1976.
43. Pittmann KA, Smyth RD, Mayol RF. Serum levels of butorphanol by radioimmuno-assay. J Pharm Sci 69:160, 1980.
44. Elliot HW, Navarro G, Nomof N. Double-blind controlled study of the pharmacologic effects of nalbuphine (En-2234A). J Med (Basel) 1:74, 1970.
45. Forrest WH, Jr. Report of the Veterans Administration Cooperative Analgesic Study: Parenteral Analgesic Bioassay of Endo 2234 A (N-Cyclobutyl-methyl-7-8-dihydro-14hydroxynormorphine). Probl Drug Depend 239:81, 1971.
46. Beaver WT, Feise GA. Comparison of the analgesic effect of intramuscular nalbuphine and morphine in patients with postoperative pain. Clin Pharmacol Therap 19:103, 1976.
47. Beaver WT, Feise GA. A comparison of the analgesic effect of intramuscular nalbuphine and morphine in patients with postoperative pain. J Pharmacol Exper Ther 204:487, 1978.

48. Beaver WT, Feise GA. Comparison of the analgesic effect of intramuscular and oral nalbuphine in patients with postoperative pain. Clin Pharmacol Therap 23:108, 1978.
49. Bikhazi GB. Comparison of morphine and nalbuphine in postoperative pediatric patients. Anesthesiology Rev 5:34, 1978.
50. Okun R. Analgesic effects of oral nalbuphine and codeine in patients with postoperative pain. Clin Pharmacol Therap 32:517, 1982.
51. Stambaugh JE. Evaluation of nalbuphine efficacy and safety in the management of advanced malignancy. Clin Pharmacol Therap 29:284, 1981.
52. Romagnoli A, Keats AS. Comparative hemodynamic effects of nalbuphine and morphine in patients with coronary artery disease. Cardiovascular Disease. Bull Texas Heart Inst 5:19, 1978.
53. Lee G, Low RI, Amsterdam EA, DeMaria AN, Huber PW, Mason DT. Hemodynamic effects of morphine and nalbuphine in acute myocardial infarction. Clin Pharmacol Therap 29: 625, 1981.
54. Lake CL, Duckworth EN, DiFazio CA, Durbin CG, Magruder MR. Cardiovascular effects of nalbuphine in patients with coronary or valvular heart disease. Anesthesiology 57: 498, 1982.
55. Romagnoli A, Keats AS. Ceiling effect for respiratory depression by nalbuphine. Clin Pharmacol Therap 27: 478, 1980.
56. Gal TJ, DiFazio CA, Moscicki J. Analgesic and respiratory depressant activity of nalbuphine: a comparison with morphine. Anesthesiology 57:367, 1982.
57. Magruder MR, Delaney RD, DiFazio CA. Reversal of narcotic-induced respiratory depression with nalbuphine hydrochloride. Anesthesiol Rev 9:34, 1982.
58. Julien RM. Effects of nalbuphine on normal and oxymorphone-depressed ventilatory response to carbon dioxide challenge. Anesthesiology 57:A320, 1982.
59. DiFazio CA, Moscicki JC, Magruder MR. Anesthetic potency of nalbuphine and interaction with morphine in rats. Anesth Analg 60:629, 1981.
60. Bluhm R, Zsigmond, EK, Winnie AP. Potentiation of opioid analgesia by H_1- and H_2-blockers. Life Sci 31:1229, 1982.
61. Jasinski DR, Mansky PA. Evaluation of nalbuphine for abuse potential. Clin Pharamcol Therap 13:78, 1972.
62. Muldoon S, Otto J, Freas W, Watson RL. The effects of morphine, nalbuphine, and butorphanol on adrenergic function in canine saphenous veins. Anesth Analg 62: 21, 1983.

114

63. Rosow CE, Miller ML, Poulsen-Burke J, Cochin J.
     Opiates and thermo-regulation in mice. III. Agonist-
     antagonists. J Pharmacol Exp Therap 220:468, 1982.
64. Magruder MR, Christofforetti R, DiFazio CA. Balanced
     anesthesia with nalbuphine hydrochloride. Anesthesiology
     Rev 7:25, 1980.
65. Fahmy NR. Nalbuphine in "balanced" anesthesia: its
     analgesic efficacy and hemodynamic effects. Anesthesiology
     53:S66, 1980.
66. Camagay IT, Gomez QJ. Balanced anesthesia with
     nalbuphine hydrochloride in pediatric patients:
     preliminary study. Philippine J Anesth 6:10, 1982.
67. Zsigmond EK. 1984. Hemodynamic effects and
     pharmacokinetics of diazepam-nalbuphine ataractanalgesia.
     Nalbuphine as a component of surgical anesthesia. (Ed.)
     Gomez QJ, New York Excerp Med ISSN.
68. Kumar Sm, Kothary SP, Zsigmond EK. Plasma free-norepinephrine
     and epinephrine concentrations following diazepam-ketamine
     induction in patients undergoing cardiac surgery. Acta
     Anaesth Scand 22:593, 1978.
69. Zsigmond EK, Tran L, Barabas E, Wang XY. Hemodynamic
     and endocrine effects of reversal of fentanyl-induced
     respiratory depression by nalbuphine. Anesthesiology
     61:    , 1984.
70. Man-Wai Lo, Juergens GP, Whitney CC. Determination
     of nalbuphine in human plasma by automated high-performance
     liquid chromatography with electrochemical detection.
     Res Com Chem Pathol Pharmacol 43:159, 1984.

KETAMINE AND PHENCYCLIDINES: TODAY AND TOMORROW
Elemer K. Zsigmond, M.D.

The introduction of intravenous barbiturates was a major
achievement in twentieth-century anesthesiology, since it
allowed a prompt induction of unconsciousness for inhalational
anesthesia without a protracted excitement period and without
the use of a face mask. The shortcomings of barbiturates,
e.g. lack of analgesia, depression of the cardiac contractility,
loss of peripheral vascular tone, histamine release and airway
obstruction were soon realized, therefore the search for
safer intravenous anesthetics continued. Although phencyclidine
(CI-395, PCP, or Sernyl) and cyclohexamine (CI-400) were
effective anesthetics, they produced psychotomimetic effects.
Their congener, 2-(0-chlorophenyl)-2-methylaminocyclohexamine,
ketamine (CI 581, Ketalar or Ketaject) produces adequate
anesthesia, analgesia and stimulation rather than depression
of cardiac contractility, increase rather than decrease in
vascular tone, no histamine release and no airway obstruction.
Drug synthesis succeeded in the production of a long-awaited,
unique analgesic-anesthetic-analeptic agent that opened a
new era in anesthesiology.

CHEMISTRY, BIODISPOSITION AND PHARMACOLOGY
Structure-activity relationship. Ketamine has an asymmetric
carbon, consequently, it has two isomers, the (-) and the
(+) form.[1,2] The structure of these isomers is shown in
Figure 1. Randomized, double-blind evaluation of the ketamine
isomers and a racemic mixture showed that (+) ketamine was a
more effective anesthetic than either the racemic mixture or
(-) ketamine, while the (-) ketamine caused a higher incidence

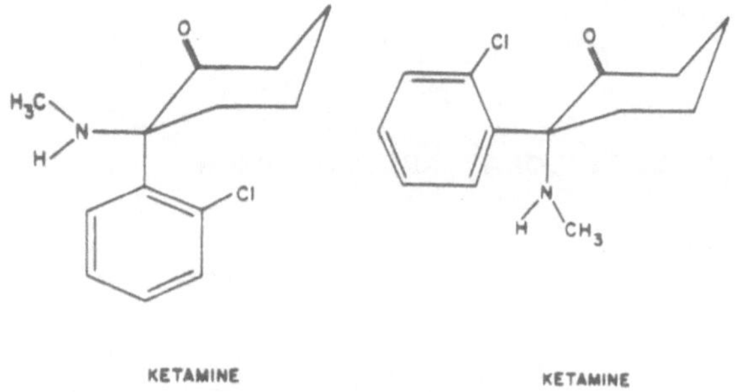

116

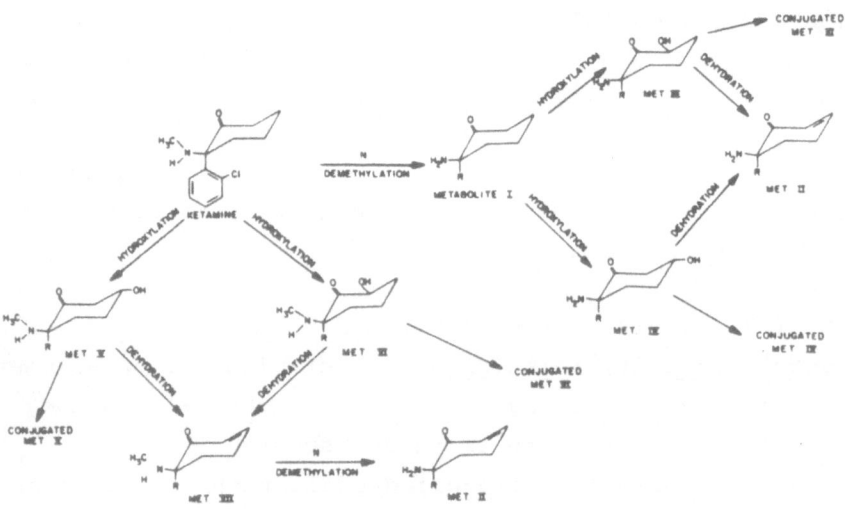

KETAMINE   KETAMINE

FIG. 1. R and S forms of ketamine.

of psychotropic response and agitation than the (+) ketamine.
Furthermore, the N-methyl (+) ketamine reaches higher
concentration in the brain tissue than the N-methyl (-)
ketamine.[3] Unfortunately the separation of enantiomers is
too expensive, therefore only the racemic form is offered
commercially.

Metabolism. Ketamine is demethylated by the hepatic P450
microsomal enzyme system to metabolite I (norketamine) which
is hydroxylated in two different positions to form metabolite
III and metabolite IV, as shown in Figure 2.

FIG. 2. Postulated biotransformation of ketamine.

These may be conjugated to glucuronides and excreted in the urine or dehydrated into metabolite II (dehydronorketamine). Its cyclohexamine ring can also be hydroxylated into metabolite V and metabolite VI. These latter products can be dehydrated to metabolite VIII.[4] Recently, the in vivo existence of metabolite II was questioned.[5] In urine, 4% unchanged ketamine and 16% hydroxylated derivatives were detected following its i.v. administration, while fecal excretion is only about 5%.[6,7]

Biodisposition and pharmacokinetics. Ketamine is similar to rapidly-acting intravenous barbiturates in its biodisposition and pharmacokinetics. It is primarily distributed to vessel-rich organs followed by its redistribution to vessel-poor organs and body fat. Typical plasma levels of ketamine vary from 9,000-26,000 ng/mL one minute after injection to 1,000 ng/mL as the patient begins to recover consciousness.[7] A logarithmic decline in plasma levels of ketamine results in a 5-15 ng/mL plasma ketamine level 24 hours after injection. The plasma levels of ketamine I and II are first detectable approximately 5 minutes after ketamine injection. Ketamine I levels at 60 minutes after injection are 245-668 ng/mL, declining to 15 ng/mL within 24 hours. Ketamine II levels decline from 515 ng/mL within 60 minutes to 13-27 ng/mL at 24 hours. Recovery from anesthesia is related to the π- and α-phases of redistribution of ketamine.[7] A three-exponential equation best approximates the ketamine pharmacokinetics.[7,8] The initial distribution half life is 7-10 min; the elimination phase, both metabolic and excretory processes, has a half life of 79 min.[7] Induction or inhibition of drug metabolizing enzymes[9,10] or a decrease in renal excretion by various drugs[11] do not alter the duration of hypnosis.[11] Halothane[12] and nitrous oxide[13] reduce the required dosage of ketamine by slowing its redistribution and metabolism. Diazepam also significantly elevates the plasma levels of ketamine.[14] Other premedications may also prolong recovery from anesthesia with ketamine.[15] Idvall et al[8] observed that intravenous infusion of ketamine at 40.0 ± 20.0 µg/kg/min maintains a plasma level of 8.8 ± 3.1 µmoles/L. Patients woke up at

2.7 ± 0.9 µmoles/L. The β-half life of ketamine in plasma
was 75 ± 9 minutes in Idvall's study. An analogue computer
model for the pharmacokinetics of ketamine after i.m. injection
in children correctly predicted the observed plasma levels.[16]

Repeated and chronic administration of ketamine to laboratory
animals[17] and to burn[18] and radiotherapy patients[19] was claimed
to lead to tolerance in contrast to our findings in thousands
of burned patients at the University of Michigan Medical Center
over a decade. We observed no tolerance or increased dose
requirements to ketamine in burned patients and in patients
who underwent repeated radiologic studies.[20]

CNS effects. The studies of Chen et al[21] first indicated
that ketamine has an anesthetic effect in mammals. It induces
coma in man accompanied by hypertonus, purposeful movements
and nystagmic gaze rather than quiet body tonus and fixed
eyeballs with small pupils as observed by Domino et al.[22]
The depression of the thalamo-neocortical pathways and
concomitant stimulation of the limbic system led to the term
"dissociative anesthesia".[23] Further studies, however, showed
excitatory activity in both the thalamus and limbic system,[24]
without clinical evidence of seizure activity.[25] Ketamine
is an anticonvulsant rather than a convulsant drug.[26]

Signs of anesthesia. Ketamine anesthesia is characterized
by blinking, staring, closing of lids, nystagmus, strabismus,
loss of lid reflex. Wide open eyelids and horizontal or
vertical nystagmus are also present. Later on, the eyeballs
become centrally fixed as in a gaze. Therefore, the eye signs
of ketamine anesthesia differ from those caused by other i.v.
and inhalational anesthetics. The difficulty in relying on
the eye-signs of anesthesia for judging adequacy of anesthesia
is one of the major concerns of anesthesiologists, preventing
its widespread use.

Coma. Ketamine induces coma in a dose dependent manner:
0.5 mg/kg ketamine i.v. provides coma for 1.5 minutes,
1 mg/kg for 5.8 minutes and 2.0 mg/kg for 10 minutes.

EEG effects. Ketamine brings about a reduction of alpha-
wave activity, no changes in beta-waves and an increase in

delta-wave amplitude. The characteristic change in EEG is a marked increase in theta-wave amplitude.

Reflexes. The gag and cough reflexes are well preserved during ketamine anesthesia. The laryngeal reflexes and swallowing also remain unaffected. Consequently, airway obstruction and/or aspiration are less likely to occur during ketamine anesthesia than during induction with other intravenous anesthetics. Aspiration of gastric content, however, did occur during ketamine anesthesia. Therefore the stomach must be emptied of propellants, air and gases before the induction of a patient suspected of having a full stomach with a nasogastric tube, preferably with an ONAT-tube.*

Intracranial pressure. Cerebral blood flow and CSF pressure are markedly and simultaneously increased by ketamine, leading to a marked rise in intracranial pressure (ICP).[27] Hence, ketamine should be avoided in patients in whom ICP rise must be avoided. As an alternative, diazepam or thiopental pretreatment should be used prior to ketamine administration.[27,28]

Analgesia. The analgesic effect of ketamine is remarkable even in low doses and outlasts coma.[29] Although ketamine was claimed to relieve only somatic pain,[23] relief of visceral pain associated with thoracic, cardiac, and abdominal surgery was confirmed at the University of Michigan by our group. Subanesthetic doses of ketamine also relieved the pain of labor.[30] Although binding of ketamine to opiate receptors was suggested,[31,32] suppression of spinal cord activity,[33,34] interferences with afferent signals in the spinoreticular tracts[35] and in the medial medullary reticular formation[36] were claimed as alternate explanations for its analgesic effect. Since ketamine inhibits cholinesterases[37,38] it was not an unexpected finding that physostigmine antagonizes the sedative and anesthetic efects of ketamine,[39,40] although other investigators were unable to observe it.[41]

*The ONAT-tube is an anti-vomiting, anti-aspiration tube manufactured by Rockway-Industries.

Emergence reactions. Volunteers who received 0.2-0.5 mg/kg
i.v. ketamine had a reduction in perception of somatic painful
stimulation with a sensation of numbness over the whole body.
Following 1.0-2.0 mg/kg i.v. doses of ketamine, the volunteers
reported weightlessness, alterations in mood, a feeling of
being suspended in space, alterations in body image, illusions
and hallucinations.[22] Although the initial reports on ketamine
underrated the incidences of hallucinations,[22,43,44] in a
double-blind study in 100 gynecologic patients an unacceptably
high incidence of adverse psychotomimetic effects was observed
following 2.0 mg/kg i.v. ketamine for induction.[44] The
incidence of bad dreams and hallucinations exceeded 80%.
Reduction in the ketamine dose to 1.5 or 1.0 mg/kg i.v. for
induction effectively reduced the incidence of emergence
reactions.[45,46] Droperidol caused no reduction in the
unpleasant dreams and hallucinations[48] but prolonged recovery.
Moreover, droperidol premedication further increased the
incidence of emergence phenomena.[47,48] Thiopental[49] and
inhalational anesthetics[50,51] may also reduce emergence
reactions.

In 1968, we observed that pretreatment with diazepam
0.2 mg/kg i.v. 8-10 minutes prior to ketamine, 2.0 mg/kg/30"
i.v. administration markedly reduced the incidence of emergence
reactions based on our working hypothesis that a limbic
suppressant, diazepam, may inhibit the limbic stimulation
caused by ketamine.[44] In another 100 patients undergoing
gynecologic procedures, 0.3 mg/kg diazepam given i.v. 10 minutes
before ketamine 2.0 mg/kg/30" i.v. induction and maintained
by ketamine i.v. drip 60 μg/kg/min and O_2 only supplemented
by succinylcholine for muscle relaxation, not only the
incidences of hallucinations and unpleasant dreams but also
visual disturbances were markedly reduced by diazepam as
compared to the placebo group.[52] The correct time interval
between diazepam and ketamine administration is essential,
since the peak effect of diazepam develops at 7-8 min as we
learned from our studies on its effect in patients undergoing
cardioversion.[53] We also found other benzodiazepines, e.g.

lorazepam, effective in reducing the psychotomimetic effect
of ketamine, but the long lasting and potentially dangerous
amnesia following its use limits its usefulness in both
in-patients and out-patients. Nonetheless, some utilize
lorazepam in their practice successfully regardless of whether
it is given   i.v. or p.o. to prevent emergence sequelae to
ketamine.[54] The new water soluble analogues of diazepam,
flunitrazepam[55] and midazolam[56] are equally effective to
prevent the emergence sequelae to ketamine. The favorable
experience with diazepam for 15 years in alleviating both the
adverse circulatory and psychotomimetic sequelae to ketamine
in thousands of cardiac, vascular, surgical, burn, abdominal
surgery, trauma and hemorrhagic shock patients favors its
continued use[52] until adequate studies on hemodynamics,
table-tilt response, organ functions, respiration and recovery
rate will become available with the newer benzodiazepines.

Cardiovascular effect. From the pharmacology of aminoketones
it was expected that ketamine causes circulatory and CNS
stimulation rather than circulatory depression in mammals
and in man.[57] Indeed, Domino, Chodoff and Corssen in 1965
clearly demonstrated that ketamine causes increases in both
systolic and diastolic blood pressures and heart rate.[22,44]
Subsequently, Zsigmond, Kelsch and Kothary[58,59] found that
the high catecholamine blood levels observed in cardiac
patients induced with ketamine based on the recommendation
of Corssen[60] were not related to the patient condition but
resulted from the sympathetic stimulation. Hence, we abandoned
ketamine for anesthetic induction in cardiac patients in 1968
and replaced it with diazepam-ketamine, since diazepam
successfully reduced the sympathetic stimulation caused by
ketamine in 40 gynecologic patients in a double-blind study.[59,61]
Repeated studies with various dose ratios of diazepam and
ketamine by Zsigmond and associates at the University of
Michigan clearly established that this circulatory stimulation
is caused by central sympathetic stimulation rather than by
adrenomedullary stimulation or by the hypoxemia that is
induced by large intravenous doses of ketamine.[62,63,64,65]

Proof for the central effect of ketamine was obtained by
Ivankovich et al,[27] who elicited the characteristic circulatory
changes induced by peripheral injection of ketamine 2.0 mg/kg/30"
i.v.using 1/20 of this dose injected directly into the
cerebral artery of the isolated and perfused hemisphere of
goats. This central "analeptic effect" of ketamine may be
utilized in hemorrhagic and septic shock.[66,67] Other effects
of ketamine on the sympathetic nervous system through
inhibition of the intraneural uptake of catecholamines[68,69]
or by the inhibition of extraneural uptake[70] or other effects
peripherally in mammals play little importance in its
circulatory effects in man.

The circulatory stimulant effect and the concomitant
increase in norepinephrine levels can be effectively antagonized
by pretreatment with 0.2-0.3 mg/kg/5 min i.v. diazepam given
8-10 min before 2.0 mg/kg/30" i.v. ketamine[62,63,64,65,71,72]
as shown in Figures 3 and 4. Although lorazepam prevents
emergence reactions, it is unable to prevent the cardiocirculatory stimulation caused by ketamine.[73] Flunitrazepam[74] and
midazolam are equally effective to diazepam.

EFFECTS OF PLACEBO-KETAMINE AND DIAZEPAM-KETAMINE
ON MEAN MAXIMUM AND MINIMUM RADIAL ARTERIAL
BLOOD PRESSURE IN NORMAL HUMAN VOLUNTEERS

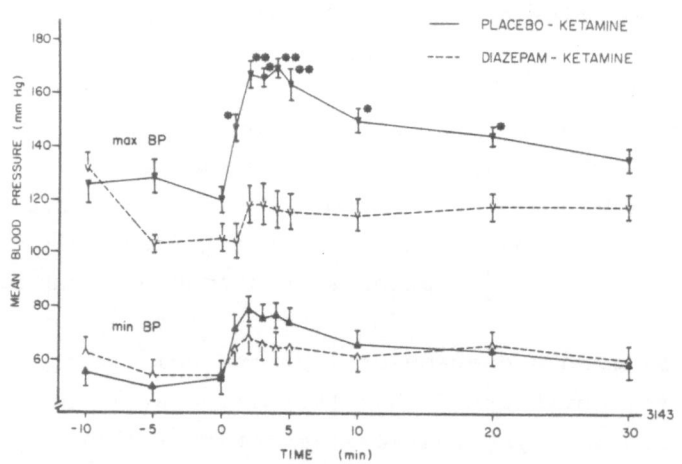

Fig. 3

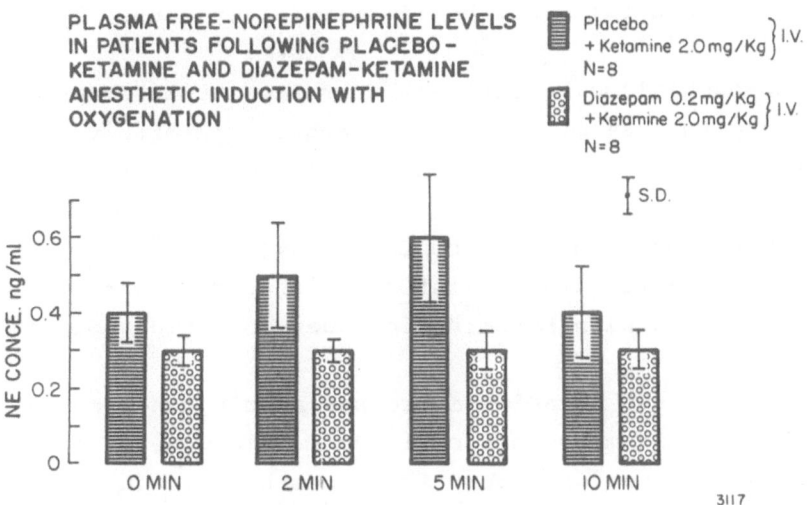

PLASMA FREE-NOREPINEPHRINE LEVELS
IN PATIENTS FOLLOWING PLACEBO-
KETAMINE AND DIAZEPAM-KETAMINE
ANESTHETIC INDUCTION WITH
OXYGENATION

Placebo
+ Ketamine 2.0 mg/Kg } I.V.
N=8

Diazepam 0.2 mg/Kg
+ Ketamine 2.0 mg/Kg } I.V.
N=8

Fig. 4

Pulmonary artery pressure is elevated by ketamine, therefore ketamine is preferably avoided in patients with decreased right ventricular reserve,[75] since ketamine increases pulmonary vascular resistance.

Cerebral blood flow is increased by ketamine that leads to an increase in cerebrospinal fluid pressure.[76,77] We succeeded in preventing this increase in cerebral blood flow and CSF pressure by pretreatment with diazepam or thiopental in neurosurgical patients.

Ventilatory effects. Ketamine causes complete apnea when given i.v. at a 2.0 mg/kg/30" rate of injection leading to arterial hypoxemia exceeding that which occurs with 0.2 mg/kg/30" rate of i.v. morphine.[62] Pretreatment with diazepam i.v. 0.3 mg/kg/30" enhances this respiratory depressant effect.[78] Reduced rate of infusion e.g. 1.0 mg/kg i.v. causes insignificant changes in Pa_{O_2} and arteriovenous oxygen differences in patients undergoing vaginal deliveries.[79] The response to hypercapnia is not altered during ketamine anesthesia.[80] Lower shunt fractions were observed during ketamine one-lung anesthesia than with halothane.[81]

Airway resistance is decreased and bronchospasm is relieved by ketamine anesthesia.[82] This effect is very likely to be related to the central sympathetic stimulation caused by ketamine.[27]

Tracheobronchial secretions are increased by ketamine necessitating the use of an antisialagogue, preferably glycopyrrolate that is void of CNS effects. Depression of laryngeal reflexes during ketamine anesthesia may develop, thereby aspiration of gastric contents may occur.[83] Gastric emptying in patients with full stomachs should be carried out prior to induction with ketamine in order to avoid aspiration pneumonitis.

Skeletal muscle. Ketamine increases muscle tone and may cause jerky, sudden movements of large muscle groups. Grimacing may indicate recovery from anesthesia. The sudden movements may resemble consciousness.[22,23,52] Despite these effects of ketamine, it has safely been used in myopathic and malignant hyperthermic patients.[84,85]

More succinylcholine is required for maintenance of muscle relaxation during ketamine anesthesia supplemented by oxygen only than during thiamylal-$N_2O:O_2$ anesthesia.[52] On the contrary, potentiation of the neuromuscular blocking effect of succinylcholine, d-tubocurarine but not that of pancuronium was reported.[86,87] More research is needed in this area.

Uterine muscle activity in pregnant uteruses may be increased if the doses exceed the analgesic doses, 0.2-0.4 mg/kg i.v. necessary for the relief of labor pain.[88] Both basal uterine tone and intensity of contractions are increased with ketamine, especially when administered during the first trimester of pregnancy. This is an ergometrine-like effect of ketamine.[89]

Effects on liver function. Healthy volunteers who received 2.0 mg/kg/30" i.v. ketamine on 2 occasions at least 2 weeks apart[90] and 156 healthy gynecologic patients who received 2.0 mg/kg/30" ketamine i.v. in a double-blind study showed no alterations in SGOT, SGPT, alkaline phosphatase, bilirubin or plasmacholinesterase.[52]

Effects on kidney function. No adverse effects of ketamine
on kidney function have been reported as yet. In 156 healthy
gynecologic patients who received 2.0 mg/kg/30" i.v. induction
with ketamine followed by ketamine i.v. drip at 60 µg/kg/min,
we observed no elevation of creatinine, no changes in urine
specific gravity or urine output.[44]

Endocrine effects. While halothane and thiopental cause
marked increases in serum free-fatty acids and blood glucose,
ketamine causes only a moderate increase in blood glucose and a
decrease in fatty acids.[91] Thyroxine levels are not altered
by ketamine, but T_3 levels are reduced.[92] No change in renin
activity during ketamine anesthesia was reported.[93] Corticosteroids
are increased by ketamine.[94]

Metabolic effects. There is an increase in metabolism
following the administration of ketamine. Increased muscle
tone and sympathetic stimulation are partly responsible for
this increase. Diazepam pretreatment reduces sympathetic
stimulation thereby the metabolic rate increase following
ketamine.

CLINICAL USES OF KETAMINE
Ketamine as a sole agent for anesthesia is usually used in
children and burn patients, while in adults most anesthesiologists
prefer the combination of diazepam with ketamine or another
benzodiazepine as pretreatment. The use of diazepam or other
benzodiazepines in children is still controversial. The fact
that ketamine produces predictable coma, amnesia and analgesia
following its i.m. administration allows its use prior to the
establishment of an intravenous line, especially in children
and in trauma patients,without the hazards of airway obstruction.

There are other contraindications to the use of ketamine:
hypertension; right or left heart failure; angina; myocardial
infarction; intracranial, thoracic or abdominal aneurysms;
cerebral trauma; intracerebral hemorrhage; increased intracranial
or intraocular pressure; thyrotoxic states; and hypermetabolic
states.

Pediatric anesthesia. Intramuscular ketamine, 5-10 mg/kg
has been widely used for diagnostic and minor surgery procedures

prior to the placement of i.v. line without endotracheal intubation.[15] Its usefulness in pediatric radiotherapy is well established.[95] For bronchoscopy[96] and for eye-examinations[97] ketamine was found to be very useful provided that adequate antisialagogue premedication is used since ketamine stimulates airway secretions.

Burn patients. Ketamine has been used daily in the Burn Unit of the University of Michigan since its introduction into anesthesia for burn dressing changes, debridements and skin grafting[98] in doses of 1.5-6.0 mg/kg i.m. A marked reduction in anesthetic morbidity and mortality in burn patients resulted from its routine use, since ketamine obviated the need for endotracheal intubation and for succinylcholine in many instances.[98] Hence the complications associated with the use of succinylcholine especially in combination with inhalational anesthetics could be avoided.[98,99] Despite reported tolerance to ketamine,[17] we were unable to substantiate it even in patients who received more than 20 ketamine administrations.[20]

Geriatric and poor-risk patients. Corssen and associates primarily have utilized ketamine in geriatric and poor-risk patients in whom other anesthetic agents and techniques were contraindicated.[23,42,60,100] Especially in patients in hemorrhagic or hypovolemic shock, hypoalbuminemia and/or electrolyte imbalance, we and others found it useful in place of halogenated anesthetic agents[101,102,103] especially in an intravenous drip. We have never noted a depression of cardiocirculatory function or maldistribution of blood flow as some investigators reported[104] in thousands of patients who were in hemorrhagic shock or hypovolemic since 1968. In severe asthmatic adults and children ketamine may be utilized as a main anesthetic agent, since it causes bronchodilation, increased compliance, and even counteracts bronchospasm occurring during halothane anesthesia.[105,106] In narcotic addicts, we have been utilizing ketamine as sole anesthetic agent since 1968 with good patient acceptance without the fear of an acute withdrawal reaction and cardiac arrhythmias in those with septic endocarditis.[20] Ketamine can be safely used in patients on bronchodilators, since it causes no sensitization of the heart to catecholamines. [107,108,109] Since ketamine can be used with 100% oxygen without N_2O supplementation, it is ideally suited for the management of patients who require high inhaled O_2 concentrations. We also managed patients with ketamine i.v. drip who had trauma to one lung and received endobronchial one-lung anesthesia or who suffered pericardial tamponade.[110]

As listed in Table 4, ketamine has a number of advantages as compared to intravenous thiamylal for the induction and maintenance of anesthesia for poor-risk patients.

Ketamine has many advantages over thiamylal in patients whose diseases contraindicate the use of intravenous rapidly acting barbiturates. These include (1) patients with congestive heart failure; (2) hypovolemic patients owing to acute hemorrhage; (3) patients with reduced cerebral blood flow (such as occlusive diseases); (4) patients in whom positional changes are required for the operation; (5) asthmatic patients; (6) patients with allergic diathesis; (7) patients in renal failure whose excretion of barbiturates is reduced; and (8) patients in hepatic failure whose metabolism of barbiturates is reduced.

Obstetrical anesthesia. Ketamine (1.0 mg/kg) causes no rise in blood pressure, no uterine vasoconstriction, and little neurobehavioral changes,[111] but 2.0 mg/kg may induce hypertension and hypertonus of the uterus[112] and neonatal depression.[113,114] The transplacental transfer of ketamine is rapid, and complete equilibration is reached between the fetal and maternal blood within minutes.[113,115,116,117,118]

Neonatal neurobehavioral studies show prolonged effects after large doses of ketamine, but minimal or no effects with 0.25 to 0.5 mg/kg doses. Ketamine in small doses (e.g., 10 mg increments each in five to ten minutes or an intravenous drip of 0.5 mg/kg/hr) maintains analgesia during obstetric procedures. It is particularly useful in bleeding patients since it causes no loss of vasomotor control and slightly stimulates the sympathetic nervous system. In emergency cesarean sections or bleeding patients for emergency surgery, one may use 0.5 to 1.0 mg/kg/1 minute for induction and 0.5 mg/kg/hr for maintenance

Table 1 Advantages of ketamine in anesthetic practice

Clinical pharmacology	Clinical practice
High therapeutic index.	Safe in poor risk patients
Rapid redistribution.	Amenable to intravenous continuous infusion.
Adequate metabolism.	Low cumulation potential.
No sustained cardiocirculatory depressant effect.	Consider using in cardiac patients.
No apparent histamine release.	Allergic response is rare.
No alteration of table tilt response.	Positional changes are not hazardous.
Stimulates central nervous system sympathetic activity.	Sudden cardiovascular collapse is unlikely.
Stimulates reflexes.	Circulatory stimulant effect, if desired.
No organ toxicity.	No hazard to patient.
Low abuse potential present.	Patient or occupational hazards negligible with restricted access to drug.

Table 2 Disadvantages of ketamine in anesthetic practice

1. Marked increase in blood pressure and heart rate.
2. High incidence of excitatory phenomena and rejection on a second occasion.
3. Difficulty in assessing anesthetic depth and the need for additional doses.
4. Increased ICP, CBF, and CSF pressure.
5. Increased metabolism.
6. Increased secretions.
7. Incidence of nausea and vomiting ranges from 15–20%.

Table 3 Recommended doses of ketamine

Management	Diazepam rate of administration	Time interval	Ketamine rate of administration
For induction	If none	-	1.0 mg/kg/30"
	0.2-0.4 mg/kg/5'	10 min	2.0 mg/kg/30"
For maintenance	If none	-	1.0 mg/kg/hr
	0.2-0.4 mg/kg/5'	10 min	1.0-2.0 mg/kg/hr
For analgesia and amnesia	0.2-0.4 mg/kg/5'	10 min	0.5-1.0 mg/kg/hr
For analgesia alone	If none	-	0.5-1.0 mg/kg/hr

When diazepam is given to counteract the side effects of ketamine, the optimum time interval, 5 to 15 minutes before ketamine intravenous administration, should be strictly observed to achieve full protection from emergence reactions.

Table 4 Comparison of ketamine and intravenous thiamylal for anesthetic induction

Site of action	Anesthetic induction agents	
	2.0 mg/kg ketamine	5.0 mg/kg thiamylal
Cardiac ejection fraction	Short moderate ↓	Prolonged severe ↓↓
Blood pressure	↑↑	↓
Peripheral vascular resistance	↑↑	↓
Cardiac output	↑↑	↓↓
Perfusion of vital organs	↑	↓
Central regulation of the circulation	↑↑	↓↓
Minute ventilation	Short severe ↓↓	Prolonged moderate ↓
Bronchial muscle tone	↓	↑
Pulmonary shunting	=	↑↑
Cerebral blood flow	↑	↓
Histamine release	=	↑

of anesthesia in combination with 50 percent N_2O or only oxygen. Ketamine caused bad dreams in 12% of 371 mothers who received ketamine 0.5-1.0 mg/kg for obstetrical delivery, while its incidence was 3% in 377 patients who received anesthetics other than ketamine.[119] Nonetheless, after the delivery, intravenous diazepam can be given to supplement ketamine analgesia and to prevent hallucinations and bad dreams.[44] Succinylcholine can be used for muscle relaxation in slightly increased doses with ketamine.[52] Pancuronium is compatible with ketamine and may prevent ketamine-induced sympathetic stimulation.[120] It must be kept in mind that ketamine may cause arterial hypoxemia in the parturient unless the dose is kept below 1.0 mg/kg.[62] The major advantages of ketamine over thiopental include the following: (1) cardiac depression does not occur; (2) sympathetic autoregulation is well maintained; and (3) no histamine release occurs.

Outpatient anesthesia. Ketamine 0.5 mg/kg i.v. with $N_2O:O_2$ gave adequate anesthesia for laparoscopy and was favored over methohexital 1.0 mg/kg i.v.[48] Barbiturate (pentobarbital 1.5 mg/kg i.m. or i.v.) reduces the incidence of emergence reactions but delays recovery.[121] The racemic ketamine alone in a total dose of 5.4 mg. i.v. caused 85% dreams and 35% refusal of subsequent ketamine anesthesia in patients who underwent curettage.[122] In a national study evaluating the efficacy and safety of low-dose intravenous (mini-drip) ketamine hydrochloride and concurrent intravenous diazepam in the induction and maintenance of balanced anesthesia, 70% of patients had a perfect recovery score of 10 and short unmeaningful emergence reactions were reported in only 0.9% of the patients studied, considerably less than in studies to which comparisons were made in 244 patients who received 0.5 to 2.46 mg/kg ketamine and 0.07 to 0.5 mg/kg diazepam concurrently for induction and 0.08 to 8.75 mg/min of ketamine.[123] Pretreatment with diazepam 8-15 min prior to ketamine induction hourly almost completely prevented circulatory and psychotomimetic adverse effects in a double-blind study done in 100 outpatients undergoing gynecologic procedures,[44,61] hence this is our preferred technique at the present time. The introduction of midazolam will provide a water-soluble alternative to diazepam.

Orthopedic surgery. Short procedures, cast applications, reductions of fractures, and dislocations can be executed using ketamine anesthesia without endotracheal intubation and general anesthesia in a preoxygenated patient who, following the emptying of his stomach, has no more food intake, but receives an antisialagogue premedication and cimetidine-alkaline combination.

Ophthalmologic and ENT surgery. Ketamine may be useful for certain diagnostic procedures, for eye examinations in children, and as a sole anesthetic in combination with muscle relaxants and $N_2O:O_2$ especially in geriatric patients with multiple systemic diseases. An i.v. drip of 0.5 mg/kg/hour following 0.1 mg/kg diazepam may be used in geriatric patients for cataract surgery. In major and long-lasting ENT surgery performed on patients in poor physical condition or who are chronic alcoholics and smokers, the diazepam-ketamine combination can be used with an advantage over other agents.

Abdominal surgery. It is evident that the patients who received ketamine for visceral abdominal surgery have had no unpleasant recall or pain, although it was thought that the drug caused only somatosensory analgesia.[44]

Plastic and reconstructive surgery. We have utilized diazepam-ketamine for the supplementation of local infiltration anesthesia and regional anesthesia without adverse circulatory and psychotomimetic sequelae.*

Cardiothoracic anesthesia. Although Corssen et al[60] recommended ketamine as a sole anesthetic agent for cardiac surgery, it may be deleterious, since it increases heart rate, blood pressure, rate-pressure product, pulmonary vascular resistance and increased left and right ventricular work.[124] In cardiac patients that require a high sympathetic tone for maintenance of vital tissue perfusion, e.g. cardiac tamponade, constrictive pericarditis or who undergo one-lung anesthesia, ketamine may be used in preference to other agents, because of the sympathetic stimulation and maintenance of intact hypoxic bronchomotor response, thereby

*Zsigmond, E.K. and Dingman, O.P.: Personal Communication 1972.

132

preventing increased shunting.[110] In cardiac patients undergoing tricuspid valvulotomy because of endocarditis caused by drug addiction, ketamine for induction and maintenance has been our choice since 1968.

For valvular surgery other than tricuspid valvulotomy, we have been utilizing 0.3-0.4 mg/kg/5min diazepam followed 8-15 min later by 1.0-2.0 mg/kg/30" ketamine for induction and fentanyl or ketamine for maintenance of anesthesia since 1968. Our first five years' experience showed that this anesthetic technique is safer than other anesthetic techniques employed.[125] Further studies on hemodynamics and catecholamines conducted at the University of Michigan in cardiac patients induced with ketamine showed no significant increase in rate-pressure product and plasma catecholamines following induction with this technique.[126,127] In contrast to morphine, which causes unacceptably high increase in histamine and catecholamine levels, diazepam-ketamine followed by ketamine i.v. drip was well tolerated.[128] Others confirmed the adequacy of diazepam-ketamine-nitrous oxide anesthesia for coronary bypass surgery.[129,130,131]

Neurosurgical anesthesia. We have utilized diazepam-ketamine-nitrous oxide anesthetic induction in neurosurgical patients placed into the sitting position, since diazepam-ketamine in contrast to placebo-ketamine caused no depression of the table-tilt response that is essential for the maintenance of normal systemic blood pressure and cerebral blood flow.[132] If an increase in intracranial pressure is to be avoided e.g. brain tumor patients, we utilize a sleep-inducing dose of thiopental prior to ketamine administration based on the work on canine cerebral blood flow and metabolism.[27,28]

CONCLUSIONS

Ketamine is an anesthetic agent with unique properties: analgesic in low doses; amnesic and anesthetic in higher doses; and analeptic in very high doses with great safety margin. Diazepam prevents the disturbing circulatory and emergence reactions to ketamine, when given in the proper dose as a pretreatment intravenously at least 10 minutes before ketamine. Other benzodiazepines, flunitrazepam and midazolam are equally

effective to diazepam. The use of high doses of ketamine is
justified only in a few clinical situations. Moderate doses
of ketamine, 0.5-1.0 mg/kg/30" are adequate for induction of
anesthesia, amnesia and analgesia but may require muscle
relaxants for atonia necessary for the conduct of surgery.
Low doses 0.2-0.5 mg/kg/30" induce adequate analgesia for labor,
minor surgery, diagnostic procedures and minor radiologic
procedures. Since ketamine provides complete anesthesia with
amnesia and analgesia, 100% oxygen may be utilized in patients
in whom N_2O is contraindicated. The lack of organotoxicity
and teratogenecity in combination with its safety with regard
to occupational exposure and/or addiction make it a widely
acceptable anesthetic and/or analgesic agent. Ketamine is
amenable to intravenous drip administration for even long and
repeated surgical procedures with efficiency and safety. Based
on the available pharmacokinetics of ketamine, the pragmatic
approach to the use of ketamine should be its administration
in an intravenous drip.

EPILOGUE

Based on the pharmacochemical studies with amino-ketones[57]
and findings of White with (+) ketamine,[3] the (+) ketamine
isomer would be preferable to the racemic mixture because of
the lower side-effect liability. Unfortunately, the chemical
separation of (+) ketamine from the racemic mixture is not cost
effective, hence it is available only for a few researchers.
Of the many congeners of ketamine, no one was found superior
to ketamine as yet. Hopefully, drug research will succeed in
the production of a ketamine-derivative without the emergence
reaction and circulatory side-effect liability.

Diazepam and other benzodiazepines are very effective and
safe in preventing the side effects with ketamine. Now, two
water-soluble benzodiazepines are available to replace diazepam
and thereby prevent the complications induced by diazepam e.g.
thrombophlebitis and burning pain on injection.Hopefully, midazolam will share the advantages of diazepam in anesthetic practice.
Further research is needed in this field.

134

REFERENCES

1. Stevens CL. Belgium Pat #634,208 in 1963 corresponding to Parke-Davis U.S. Pat #3,254,124 in 1966.
2. Hudyma TW, Holmes SW,Hooper IR. Chem Abst 75:118119X 1971 corresponding to Bristol-Myers German Pat #2,062,620 in 1971.
3. White PF, Ham J, Way WL et al. Pharmacology of ketamine isomers in surgical patients. Anesthesiology 52:231,1980.
4. Chang T, Glazko AJ. Biotransformation and disposition of ketamine. Int Anesth Clinic 19:157, 1974.
5. Adams JD, Baillie TA, Trevor AJ et al. Studies on the bio-transformation of ketamine—identification of metabolites produced in vitro from rat liver microsomal preparations. Biomed Mass Spectr 8:527, 1981.
6. Wieber J, Gugler R, Hengstmann JH et al. Pharmacokinetics of ketamine in man. Anaesthesist 24:260, 1975.
7. Domino EF, Zsigmond EK, Domino LE et al. Plasma levels of ketamine and two of its metabolites in surgical patients using a gas chromatographic mass fragmentographic assay. Anesth Analg 61:87, 1982.
8. Idvall J, Ahlgren I, Aronsen KF et al. Ketamine infusions: pharmacokinetics and clinical effects. Brit J Anaesth 51:1167, 1979.
9. Cohen ML, Trevor AJ. On the cerebral accumulation of ketamine and the relationship between metabolism of the drug and its pharmacological effects. J Pharmacol Exp Ther 189:351, 1974.
10. Marietta MP, White PF, Pudwill CR et al. Biodisposition of ketamine in the rat: self-induction of metabolism. J Pharmacol Exp Ther 196:536, 1976.
11. Letajet J, Bouletreau P, Cilles YD et al. Kétamine et insuffisuance rénale. Anesth Analg (Paris) 29:261, 1972.
12. White PF, Marietta MP, Pudwill CR et al. Effects of halothane anesthesia on the biodisposition of ketamine in rats. J Pharmacol Exp Ther 196:545, 1976.
13. Wessels JV, Allen GW, Slogoff S. The effect of nitrous oxide on ketamine anesthesia. Anesthesiology 39:382, 1973.
14. Domino EF, Zsigmond EK, Smith RE. Diazepam on the pharmacokinetics of ketamine in man. Excerp Med ICS 533:1237, 1980.
15. Wyant GM. Intramuscular ketalar (CI-581) in pediatric anesthesia. Can Anaesth Soc J 18:72, 1971.
16. Torr G, Stella L. Distribution of ketamine following i.v. and i.m. administration. Minerva Anesthesiol 43:413, 1977.
17. Marietta MP, White PF, Pudwill CR et al. Biodisposition of ketamine in the rat: self-induction of metabolism. J Pharmacol Exp Ther 196:536, 1976.
18. Demling RH, Ellerbee S, Jarrett F. Ketamine anesthesia for tangential excision of burn eschar: a burn unit procedure. J Trauma 18:269, 1978.
19. Cronin MM, Bousfield JD, Hewitt EB et al. Ketamine anesthesia for radiotherapy in small children. Anesthesia 27:135, 1972.
20. Lieding KR, Zsigmond EK. Personal Communications, 1974.

21. Chen G, Ensor CR, Bohner B. The neuropharmacology of 2-(0-chlorophenyl)-2-methylaminocyclohexanone hydrochloride. J Pharmacol Exp Ther 152:332, 1966.
22. Domino EF, Chodoff P, Corssen G. Pharmacologic effects of CI-581, a new dissociative anesthetic, in man. Clin Pharmacol Exp Ther 6:279, 1965.
23. Corssen G, Miyasaka M, Domino EF. Changing concepts in pain control during surgery: Dissociative anesthesia with CI-581. Anesth Analg (Cleve) 47:746, 1968.
24. Kayama Y, Iwama K. The EEG, evoked potentials and single-unit activity during ketamine anesthesia in cats. Anesthesiology 36:316, 1972.
25. Corssen G, Little SC, Tavakoli M. Ketamine and epilepsy. Anesth Analg (Cleve) 53:319, 1974.
26. Reder BS, Trapp LD, Troutman KC. Ketamine suppression of chemically induced convulsions in the two-day-old white leghorn cockerel. Anesth Analg 59:406, 1980.
27. Ivankovich AD, Miletich DJ, Reimann C, Albrecht RF, Zahed B. Cardiovascular effects of centrally administered ketamine in goats. Anesth Analg 53:924, 1974.
28. Dawson B, Michenfelder JD, Theye RA. Effects of ketamine on canine cerebral blood flow and metabolism: modification by prior administration of thiopental. Anesth Analg 50:443, 1971.
29. Bjarnesen W, Corssen G. CI-581: A new non-barbiturate short-acting anesthetic for surgery in burns. Mich Med 66:177, 1967.
30. Aguado-Matorras A, Nalda-Felipe MA, Vidal-Macho J et al. Experiencia personal de 300 casos de DI-581 (ketamina) en anestesiología. Rev Esp Anestesiol Réanim 17:302, 1970.
31. Vincent JP, Corey D, Kamenka JM et al. Interaction of phencyclidines with the muscarinic and opiate receptors in the central nervous system. Brain Res 152:176, 1978.
32. Smith DJ, Westfall DP, Adams JD et al. Ketamine interacts with opiate receptors as an agonist. Anesthesiology 53:S5, 1980.
33. Conseiller C, Benoist JM, Hamann KF et al. Effects of ketamine (CI-581) on cell responses to cutaneous stimulations in laminae IV and V in cat's dorsal horn. Eur J Pharmacol 18:346, 1972.
34. Kitahata LM, Taub A, Kosaka Y. Lamina-specific suppression of dorsal-horn unit activity by ketamine hydrochloride. Anesthesiology 38:4, 1973.
35. Sparks DL, Corssen G, Sides J et al. Ketamine-induced anesthesia: Neural mechanisms in rhesus monkeys. Anesth Analg 52:288, 1973.
36. Ohtani M, Kikuchi H, Kitahata LM et al. Effects of ketamine on nociceptive cells in the medial medullary reticular formation of the cat. Anesthesiology 51:414, 1979.
37. Flynn JS, Zsigmond EK. The effect of ketamine (Ketalar, CI-581) on human plasma cholinesterase. (Abstract) Clin Pharmacol Therap 11:300, 1970.

136

38. Cohen ML, Chan SL, Bhargava HN et al. Inhibition of mammalian brain acetylcholinesterase by ketamine. Biochem Pharmacol 23:1647, 1974.
39. Balmer HGR, Wyte SR. Antagonism of ketamine by physostigmine. Br J Anaesth 49:510, 1977.
40. Lawrence D, Livingston A. The effect of physostigmine and neostigmine on ketamine anaesthesia and analgesia. Br J Pharmacol 67:426, 1979.
41. Drummond JC, Brebner J, Galloon S et al. A randomized evaluation of the reversal of ketamine by physostigmine. Can Anaesth Soc J 26:288, 1979.
42. Oduntan SA, Gool RY. Clinical trial of ketamine (CI-581). Can Anaesth Soc J 17:411, 1970.
43. Moore J, McNabb TG, Dundee JW. Preliminary report on ketamine in obstetrics. Br J Anaesth 43:779, 1971.
44. Kothary SP, Zsigmond EK. A double-blind study of the effective antihallucinatory doses of diazepam prior to ketamine anesthesia. Clin Pharmacol Ther 21:108, 1977.
45. Ellingson A, Haram K, Sagen N. Ketamine and diazepam as anesthesia for forceps delivery. A comparative study. Acta Anaesth Scan 21:37, 1977.
46. Krantz ML. Ketamine in obstetrics: Comparison with methoxy-flurane. Anesth Analg 53:890, 1974.
47. Erbguth PH, Reiman B, Klein RL. The influence of chlorpromazine, diazepam and droperidol on emergence from ketamine. Anesth Analg 51:693, 1972.
48. Figallo EM, Casali H, McKenzie R et al. Ketamine as the sole anaesthetic agent for laparoscopic sterilization. Br J Anaesth 49:1159, 1977.
49. Liang HS, Liang HG. Minimizing emergence phenomena: Subdissociative dosage of ketamine in balanced surgical anesthesia. Anesth Analg 54:312, 1975.
50. Bidwai AV, Stanley TH, Graves CL et al. The effects of ketamine on cardiovascular dynamics during halothane and enflurane anesthesia. Anesth Analg 54:588, 1975.
51. El-Naggar M, Kintanar D, Rodenas J et al. Ketamine as an induction agent and an adjunct to nitrous oxide-oxygen curare anesthesia sequence. Anesthesiol Rev 4:10, 1975.
52. Zsigmond EK, Domino EF. Clinical pharmacology and current uses of ketamine. In Aldrete JA, Stanley TH: Trends in intravenous anesthesia. Symposia Specialists, Miami, 1980, pp283-330.
53. Zsigmond EK. Causes of ventricular arrhythmias. JAMA 221:712, 1972.
54. Lilburn JK, Dundee JW, Nair SG et al. Ketamine sequelae: Evaluation of the ability of various premedicants to attenuate its psychic actions. Anaesthesia 33:307, 1978.
55. De Castro J. The use of ketamine and RD5-4200 (flunitrazepam) in 1/100 ratio in i.v. subvigile anesthesia. Ars Medici 8:1287, 1972.
56. White PF. Unpublished data in White PF, Way WL, Trevor AJ. Ketamine - its pharmacology and therapeutic uses.

57. Nador K, Porszasz J. Pharmacologic and pharmochemical studies with β-aminoketones, Arzneim Forsch 8:313, 1958.
58. Zsigmond EK, Kelsch RC, Kothary SP. Plasma free norepinephrine concentration during induction with ketamine. Rev Bras Anesth 22:443, 1972.
59. Zsigmond EK. Comment on paper of Corssen GC: Ketamine in the anesthetic management of asthma patients. Anesth Analg 51:595, 1972.
60. Corssen GC, Allarde R, Brosch F, Arbenz G. Ketamine as the sole anesthetic in open-heart surgery: A preliminary report. Anesth Analg 49:1025, 1970.
61. Zsigmond EK, Kothary SP, Martinez OA, Kelsch RC. Diazepam for prevention of the rise in plasma catecholamines caused by ketamine. Abstract. Clin Pharmacol Therap 15:223, 1973.
62. Zsigmond EK, Matsuki A, Kothary SP, Jallad M. Arterial hypoxemia caused by intravenous ketamine. Anesth Analg 55:311, 1976.
63. Zsigmond EK. Ataract-analgesic mixtures: Diazepam-ketamine. Excerp Med ICS 347:136, 1974.
64. Zsigmond EK, Kothary SP, Martinez OA, Matsuki A. Circulatory and endocrine effects of ataract-analgesia with diazepam-ketamine. Excerp Med ICS 330:335, 1974.
65. Kothary SP, Zsigmond EK, Matsuki A. Antagonism of the ketamine-induced rise in plasma free-norepinephrine, blood pressure and pulse rate by intravenous diazepam. Clin Pharmacol Therap 17:238, 1975.
66. Wong DHW, Jenkins LC. The cardiovascular effects of ketamine in hypotensive states. Can Anaesth Soc J 22:339, 1975.
67. Longnecker DE, Sturgill BC. Influence of anesthetic agents on survival following hemorrhage. Anesthesiology 45:516, 1976.
68. Byrne AJ, Healy TEJ, Tomlinson DR. The effects of ketamine on noradrenergic transmission and the response to noradrenaline in rat smooth muscle. Br J Pharmacol 67:462, 1979.
69. Nedergaard OA. Cocaine-like effect of ketamine on vascular adrenergic neurons. Eur J Pharmacol 23:153, 1973.
70. Lundy PM, Gowdey CW, Colhoun EH. The actions of ketamine on vascular smooth muscle. Arch Int Pharmacodyn Ther 220:213, 1976.
71. Zsigmond EK, Kothary SP, Martinez OA et al. Diazepam for prevention of the rise in plasma catecholamines caused by ketamine. Clin Pharmacol Therap 15:223, 1974.
72. Kumar SM, Kothary SP, Zsigmond EK et al. Plasma free norepinephrine and epinephrine concentrations following diazepam-ketamine induction in patients undergoing cardiac surgery. Acta Anaesth Scand 22:593, 1978.
73. Lilburn JK, Moore J, Dundee JW. Attempts to attenuate the cardiostimulatory effects of ketamine. Anaesthesia 32:449, 1978.

74. Tarnow J, Hess W. Flunitrazepam - Pretreatment for alleviation of ketamine side effects. Anaesthesist 28:468, 1979.
75. Tarnow J, Hess W, Schmidt D et al. Anesthetic management of patients with coronary heart disease: flunitrazepam, diazepam, ketamine, fentanyl. Anaesthesist 28:9, 1979.
76. Shapiro HM, Wyte SR, Harris AB. Ketamine anesthesia in patients with intracranial pathology. Br J Anaesth 44:1200, 1972.
77. Takeshita H, Okuda Y, Sari A. The effects of ketamine on cerebral circulation and metabolism in man. Anesthesiology 36:69, 1972.
78. Zsigmond EK, Kothary SP, Matsuki A, Flynn K. Comparison of the effect of ketamine with other narcotic-analgesics on arterial blood gases in man. Excerp Med ICS 387: 170, 1976.
79. Maduska AL, Hajghassemali M. Arterial blood gases in mother and infants during ketamine anesthesia for vaginal delivery. Anesth Analg 57:121, 1978.
80. Soliman MG, Brinale GF, Kuster G. Response to hypercapnia under ketamine anaesthesia. Canad Anaesth Soc J 22: 486, 1975.
81. Lumb PD, Silvay G, Weinreich AI et al. A comparison of the effects of continuous ketamine infusion and halothane on oxygenation during one-lung anesthesia in dogs. Can Anaesth Soc J 26:394, 1979.
82. Corssen G, Gutierrez J, Reves JG et al. Ketamine in the anesthetic management of asthmatic patients. Anesth Analg 51:588, 1972.
83. Taylor PA, Towey RM. Depression of laryngeal reflexes during ketamine anesthesia. Br Med J 2:688, 1971.
84. Wadhwa RK, Tantisira B. Parotidectomy in a patient with a family history of hyperthermia. Anesthesiology 40: 191, 1974.
85. Zsigmond EK. Malignant hyperthermia with subsequent uneventful general anesthesia. Anesth Analg 50:1111, 1971.
86. Amaki Y, Nagashima H, Radnay PA et al. Ketamine interaction with neuromuscular blocking agents in the phrenic nerve-hemidiaphragm preparation of the rat. Anesth Analg 57:238, 1978.
87. Johnston RR, Miller RD, Way WL. The interaction of ketamine with d-tubocurarine, pancuronium, and succinylcholine in man. Anesth Analg 53:496, 1974.
88. Marx GF, Hwang HS, Chandra P. Postpartum uterine pressures with different doses of ketamine. Anesthesiology 50:163, 1979.
89. Oats JN, Vasey OP, Waldron BA. Effects of ketamine on the pregnant uterus. Br J Anaesth 51:1163, 1979.
90. Zsigmond EK, Domino EF, Goulet, JR. Ketamine in the hepatic function in healthy prisoner volunteers. Excerp Med ICS 533:51, 1980.

91. Kaniaris P, Lekakis D, Kykoniatis M et al. Serum free fatty acid and blood sugar levels in children under halothane, thiopentone, and ketamine anaesthesia. Can Anaesth Soc J 22:509, 1975.
92. Matsuki A, Shiga T, Sanuki K et al. Reduced triiodothyronine levels during and following ketamine-N_2O anesthesia in man. JPN J Anaesth 25:373, 1976.
93. Miller ED, Gianfagna W, Ackerly JA et al. Converting-enzyme activity and pressor response to angiotensin I and II in the rat awake and during anesthesia. Anesthesiology 50:88, 1979.
94. Oyama T, Matsumoto F, Kudo T. Effects of ketamine on adrenocortical function in man. Anesth Anlag 49:697, 1970.
95. Bennett JA, Bullimore JA. The use of ketamine hydrochloride anaesthesia for radiotherapy in young children. Br. J Anaesth 45:197, 1973.
96. Barson PK, Scott ML, Lawson NW et al. Ketamine for bronchoscopy of children. South Med J 67:1403, 1974.
97. Adams A. Ketamine in pediatric ophthalmic practice. Anesthesia 28:212, 1973.
98. Bjarnesen W, Corssen, G. CI-581: A new non-barbiturate short-acting anesthetic for surgery in burns. Mich Med 66:1177, 1967.
99. Wilson R, Nichols R, McCoy N. Dissociative anesthesia with CI-581 in burned children. Anesth Analg 46:719, 1967.
100. Vaughan RW, Stephen CR. Abdominal and thoracic surgery in adults with ketamine, nitrous-oxide and d-tubocurarine. Anesth Analg 53:271, 1974.
101. Peter K, van Ackern K, Frey B et al. Die Wirkung verschiedener Narkotika auf Herz und Kreislauf bei der Narkoseeinleitung im franhen Hämorrhägischen Schock. Z Prakt Anaesth 7:263, 1972.
102. Bond AC, Davies CK. Ketamine and pancuronium for the shocked patient. Anesthesia 29:59, 1974.
103. Chasapakis G, Kekis N, Sakkalis C et al. Use of ketamine and pancuronium for anaesthesia for patients in hemorrhagic shock. Anesth Analg 52:282, 1973.
104. Waxman K, Shoemaker WC, Lippmann M. Cardiovascular effects of anesthetic induction with ketamine. Anesth Analg 59: 355, 1980.
105. Betts GK, Parkin CE. Use of ketamine in an asthmatic child: a case report. Anesth Analg 50:420, 1971.
106. Fischer MM. Ketamine hydrochloride in severe bronchospasm. Anesthesia 32:771, 1977.
107. Ivankovich AD, El-Etr AA, Janeczko GF et al. The effects of ketamine and of Innovar anesthesia on digitalis tolerance in dogs. Anesth Analg 54:106, 1975.
108. Idvall J, Ahlgren I, Aronsen KF et al. Ketamine infusions: Pharmacokinetics and clinical effects. Br J Anaesth 51: 1167, 1979.
109. Dowdy EG, Kaya K. Studies of the mechanism of cardiovascular responses to CI-581. Anesthesiology 29:931, 1968.
110. Silvay G, Weinrich A, Lumb P et al. Continuous ketamine for one-lung anesthesia as an alternative to halothane. Excerp Med ICS 452:140, 1978.

111. Hodgkinson R, Marx GF, Kim SS et al. Neonatal neurobehavioral tests following vaginal delivery under ketamine, thiopental and extradural anesthesia. Anesth Analg 56:548, 1977.
112. Galloon S. Ketamine for obstetric delivery. Anesthesiology 44:522, 1976.
113. Little B, Chang T, Chucot L et al. Study of ketamine as an obstetric agent. Am J Obstet Gynecol 113:247, 1972.
114. Meer FM, Downing JW, Coleman AJ. An intravenous method of anesthesia for caesarean section, II Ketamine. Br J Anaesth 45:191, 1973.
115. Moore F, McNabb TG, Dundee JW. Preliminary report on ketamine in obstetrics. Br J Anaesth 43:779, 1971.
116. Janeczko GF, El-Etr AA, Younes S. Low-dose ketamine anesthesia for obstetrical delivery. Anesth Analg 53: 829, 1974.
117. Cosmi EV. 1976. Drugs, anesthetics, and the fetus. In: Scarpelli, EM and Cosmi EV (eds); Reviews in Perinatal Medicine Vol I University Park Press, Baltimore, p 191.
118. Cosmi EV. Effeti della ketamina sulla madre e sul feto. Studio sperimentale e clinico Minerva Anesthesiol 43: 379, 1977b.
119. Sechzer PH. Dreams with low-dose ketamine in obstetrical patients. Curr Therap Res 35:396, 1984.
120. Matsuki A, Zsigmond EK, Kelsch RC, Kothary SP, Martinez OA. The effect of pancuronium bromide on plasma nor-epinephrine concentration during ketamine induction. Rev Bras Anest 24:590, 1974.
121. Figallo EM, McKenzie R, Tantisira B et al. Anesthesia for dilation, evacuation, and curettage in outpatients. A comparison of subanaesthetic doses of ketamine and sodium methohexitone-nitrous oxide anaesthesia. Can Anaesth Soc J 24:110, 1977.
122. White PF, Ham J, Way WL et al. Pharmacology of ketamine isomers in surgical patients. Anesthesiology 52:231, 1980.
123. Fontenot J, et al. Efficacy and safety of low dose intravenous diazepam in the induction and maintenance of balanced anesthesia. Clin Pharmacol Therap 31:225, 1982.
124. Domino EF, Zsigmond EK. 1980. Pharmacokinetics of ketamine in man in relation to its circulatory effects. In ketamine and the cardiovascular system, Ed:. Langrehr., Excerp Med, Amsterdam-Geneva-Princeton, pp 20-29.
125. Zsigmond EK, Kothary SP, Matsuki A, Martinez O. Atara-analgesia mixtures: diazepam-ketamine. Excerp Med ICS 347:136, 1974.
126. Kumar SM, Kothary SP, Zsigmond EK. Plasma free nor-epinephrine and epinephrine concentrations following diazepam-ketamine induction in patients undergoing cardiac surgery. Acta Anesth Scand 22:593, 1978.

127. Jackson APF, Dhadphale PR, Callaghan ML. Haemodynamic studies during induction of anaesthesia for open-heart surgery using diazepam and ketamine. Br J Anaesth 50: 375, 1978.
128. Zsigmond EK, Martinez OA. Plasma epinephrine and nor-epinephrine levels during induction of morphine anesthesia in cardiac surgical patients. Rev Bras Anest 24:220, 1974.
129. Dhadphale PR, Jackson APF, Alseri S. Comparison of anesthesia with diazepam and ketamine vs. morphine in patients undergoing heart-valve replacement. Anesthesiology 51:200, 1979.
130. Hatano S, Keane DM, Boggs RE et al. Diazepam-ketamine anesthesia for open-heart surgery - a micro-mini drip administration technique. Can Anaesth Soc J 23:648, 1976.
131. Reves JG, Lell WA, McCracken LE et al. Comparison of morphine and ketamine. Anesthetic techniques for coronary surgery; a randomized study. South Med J 71:33, 1978.
132. Zsigmond EK, Kothary SP. Double-blind evaluation of the circulatory response to 60° table-tilt with diazepam-ketamine and placebo-ketamine anesthesia. Excerp Med ICS 452: 58, 1978.

THE ADULT RESPIRATORY DISTRESS SYNDROME: MECHANISMS AND MANAGEMENT

GUY A. ZIMMERMAN, M.D.

The term "adult respiratory distress syndrome", abbreviated ARDS, was coined less than 20 years ago to describe adult patients with a specific form of acute respiratory failure (1). As implied by the name, ARDS is a syndrome characterized by a group of clinical and pathophysiologic features which indicate severe lung injury that results from a variety of underlying disease processes. The key pathophysiologic feature that differentiates ARDS from other forms of acute respiratory failure in adults is diffuse injury to the alveolar capillary membrane (2). The injury can result from insults delivered via the airway (as in gastric acid aspiration or diffuse bacterial pneumonia), via the bloodstream (as in ARDS associated with gram negative bacteremia, or endotoxemia, resulting from an infectious focus distant from the lung), or via both routes. There is no single clinical feature that defines the syndrome of ARDS. Furthermore, a laboratory test that identifies diffuse alveolar capillary injury, and differentiates it from other disease processes, does not exist. Therefore the syndrome is recognized by a constellation of clinical and pathophysiologic findings (1,3) (Table 1). Each of the features listed in Table 1 can occur in association with other causes of acute respiratory failure, but together they define the clinical syndrome of ARDS. In addition to the classic findings listed in Table 1, pulmonary hypertension is a common feature in patients with this syndrome (16,17).

The characteristic clinical features, and abnormalities of gas exchange and lung mechanics in ARDS, have been extensively reviewed in several recent monographs (3-6) and will not be discussed here. The remainder of this outline will discuss features of the syndrome that have been recognized recently and are likely to influence our concept of this disease process in the future.

144

Table 1

CRITERIA FOR RECOGNITION OF ARDS

1. An underlying disease process associated with diffuse alveolar capillary injury.
2. Hypoxemia refractory to supplemental oxygen.
3. Decreased lung compliance.
4. Diffuse lung infiltrates on the chest radiograph, not due to chronic pulmonary disease.
5. Normal or low pulmonary capillary hydrostatic pressure, usually estimated by the pulmonary capillary wedge pressure.

Natural History: Originally, the course of ARDS was described as: 1) an event that likely initiated diffuse lung injury, such as gram negative septicemia or multiple trauma with shock, 2) a latent period of 12-72 hours, 3) the rapid development of severe respiratory failure, and 4) death within a short interval for many patients (1,2). Two recent reports confirm that the majority of patients who develop the syndrome do so within 72 hours of the original insult, when a finite insult can be defined (7,8). Direct injuries to the lung, such as massive gastric acid aspiration or noxious gas inhalation, may cause the syndrome to develop within a few hours (7). In contrast, in some patients (especially those with diffuse bacterial pneuemonia or indolent nonpulmonary infections without obvious bacteremia) the syndrome may develop over several days. This indicates that the natural history of the syndrome may vary depending on the underlying disease process and potentially other features, such as iatrogenic manipulations.

In contrast to earlier years, patients tend to survive longer, with a median survival in one recent report of 13.3 days after onset of the syndrome (7). Despite this the mortality rate has not improved since the syndrome was described (see below).

Patients At Risk: ARDS has been reported to be consequence of many
different underlying disease processes (4,7,8,25). However, a
relatively small number of insults commonly predispose to the
development of the syndrome. These include gastric acid aspiration,
diffuse infectious pneumonia, bacteremia and the "sepsis syndrome", and
shock, multiple trauma, fractures, and other conditions that require
multiple transfusions (7,8). Patients with more than one predisposing
condition are at higher risk than those with single conditions (7,8).
Some disease processes, such as disseminated intravascular coagulation,
pancreatitis, and near-drowning, are common in one report but are not
identified as predisposing conditions in others (7,8). This likely
reflects differences in the patient populations in individual medical
centers and biases in patient selection.

Pathology and Pathophysiology: Diffuse interstitial and alveolar edema,
due to increased permeability of the alveolar-capillary membrane to
water and macromolecules (including large molecular-weight dextrans and
proteins) is a hallmark of the acute phase of ARDS (2,5,9-12). For many
physicians ARDS is synonymous with acute respiratory failure secondary
to "noncardiogenic pulmonary edema" (9), although many patients with
increased-permeability pulmonary edema (12,13) do not develop all of the
features of ARDS (Table 1). Furthermore, longer survival of patients
with ARDS has clarified the fact that increased-permeability lung edema
is but one manifestation of the severe injury to the alveolar capillary
membrane that occurs in ARDS. Other abnormalities occur as well, and
the pathology and pathophysiologic features are different at various
stages of the syndrome. Recognition of this fact is important, since
management based primarily on the relief of lung edema may have little
or no utility in later stages of the syndrome.
     Bachofen and Weibel (10) have carefully studied the lungs of
patients with ARDS at various stages and confirm that pathologic
evidence for interstitial and alveolar edema predominates in the "acute
stage." The edema is due to injury to the endothelial and/or epithelial
cells of the alveolar-capillary membrane (2,10). These findings appear
to require 20 or more hours to develop in many patients (10) although
they may develop more rapidly in others (7,8). Lung edema may occur in
association with intravascular accumulation of polymorphonuclear

leukocytes, platelet-fibrin microthrombi, and interstitial accumulation of inflammatory cells (10,14,15). The increased endothelial permeability results in increased transvascular flow of water and protein out of the microvessels and into the interstitium at any level of intravascular hydrostatic pressure (12,13,21). The epithelial cell injury disrupts the alveolar barrier that is minimally permeable to water and small molecular weight molecules under normal conditions (20), and contributes to alveolar flooding (10). The accumulation of platelet-fibrin thrombi and granulocytes in the capillaries is likely a manifestation of severe endothelial cell injury (10), just as increased capillary permeability is such a manifestation. However, the accumulation of granulocytes and/or platelets in the microvasculature may also be a factor that initiates or amplifies pulmonary vascular injury (15,18,49-51).

If the patient survives for days to weeks, the "subacute phase" of ARDS (10) is characterized by alveolar septal thickening caused by proliferation of interstitial cells, infiltration of the interstitium with chronic inflammatory cells, hyperplasia of the alveolar Type II cell, and interstitial and alveolar fibrosis in some patients. Abnormalities of alveolar phospholipid composition and surfactant function occur (22). These changes likely represent an evolving pathologic response of the cells of the alveolar capillary membrane to injury; lung specimens with areas of fibrosis adjacent to alveoli flooded with edema have been observed (10,15). An important feature of the subacute phase in some patients is the development of pulmonary hypertension (16,17) that may be caused by a variety of mechanisms (18). These include obstruction of the microvasculature with granulocytes and/or platelet-fibrin thrombi (14,15), destruction of the microvascular bed with loss of capillary surface area (19), distortion of the interstitium (10) as well as vasoconstriction (16). It is also possible that pulmonary hypertension, and its relative resistance to vasodilator agents (16) in some patients with ARDS, may also be due to injury of the endothelial cells with loss of their ability to produce "relaxation factors" for the vascular smooth muscle (55), although this has not been shown in humans. The factors that influence the development of specific features (such as pulmonary fibrosis or severe pulmonary hypertension) in individual patients are unknown.

Recognition of the fact that multiple pathophysiologic mechanisms may be operative in patients with ARDS influences clinical management. For example, the administration of vasodilators may have little effect on pulmonary hypertension caused by vascular obstruction or destruction (16), but may have deleterious effects on cardiac output and gas exchange, and thus may be contraindicated in some patients. The progression of the syndrome from the acute to the subacute phase also has implications that may be important in the clinical management of the patient. For example, a patient who has survived for 2 weeks with ARDS may have markedly decreased lung compliance due to fibrosis rather than a major component of edema, and markedly increased alveolar deadspace and right ventricular dysfunction due to severe pulmonary hypertension. Recognition of these features would be essential for the optimal management of the patient in the intensive care unit or operating suite.

Complications in Other Organ Systems: Complications in other organ systems are common in patients with ARDS. With the exception of diffuse infectious pneumonia, lung contusion or inhalation injury, the disease processes that cause ARDS involve other organ systems at the onset. Involvement of multiple organ systems becomes more common in the subacute phase, due to complications of the respiratory failure and iatrogenic complications (23), and is a common cause of death at this point in the pathogenesis of the syndrome. Cardiovascular (16,17), gastrointestinal (23), renal (23), and infectious (24) complications are common. Prevention, recognition and skillful management of systemic complications is frequently the key to success or failure in the management of ARDS. It requires a team that is committed to the overall care of the patient and not simply to the manipulation of the patient's cardiopulmonary physiologic abnormalities. Progressive multiple organ system failure, including progressive respiratory failure, is frequently a complication of infection in ARDS (24).

Management

Since ARDS is a syndrome with multiple underlying etiologies, there is no specific cure for the disorder. The most important aspect of the

management is the identification of the etiologic cause and the
institution of appropriate therapy. Thus the identification and
appropriate treatment of infectious pneumonia, and infectious foci at
distant sites (intraabdominal abscess, etc.) that cause lung injury
because of bacteremia and/or endotoxemia, are paramount. Many of the
other etiologies of ARDS (7,8,25) have less specific therapies than do
bacterial infections, and are more difficult to manage in that respect.

The second major principle of management of ARDS is support of the
patient, and prevention of death due to the consequences of acute
respiratory failure. The fundamental concept is similar to that which
guides the support of patients with other forms of respiratory failure,
but is especially important in the management of ARDS: maintain adequate
oxygen delivery to the tissues by manipulation of oxygen transfer across
the lung, maintainance of blood oxygen-carrying capacity, and
manipulation of cardiac output if necessary. The adequacy of tissue
oxygen levels is assessed by clinical evaluation of the patient (mental
status, urine output, evidence for organ dysfunction due to hypoxia or
ischemia) and in many patients by monitoring mixed venous PO_2. The
mixed venous PO_2 gives no information about regional oxygenation; it is
currently thought to be an index of global oxygenation at the tissue
level, although its exact significance in critically-ill patients is
under scrutiny (26).

Our group has found the clinical application of the Fick Equation
(Figure 1) to be a useful way to emphasize the principle of support
aimed at adequate tissue oxygenation, and to keep in mind those
variables that can be most easily manipulated (27).

A third major principle in the management of ARDS is the
recognition and treatment of complications (see above), and careful
overall care of the patient, including nutritional support (46).

Specific Aspects of Supportive Management of ARDS: Several aspects of
the supportive management of patients with ARDS will be briefly
discussed. Although the technology has changed in the last 14 years,
the fundamental aspects are not substantially different from those
discussed in the original review of the management of this disorder
(28).

FIGURE 1

APPLICATION OF THE FICK EQUATION TO THE MANAGEMENT OF SEVERE RESPIRATORY FAILURE (INADEQUATE DELIVERY OF O_2 TO BODY CELLS)*

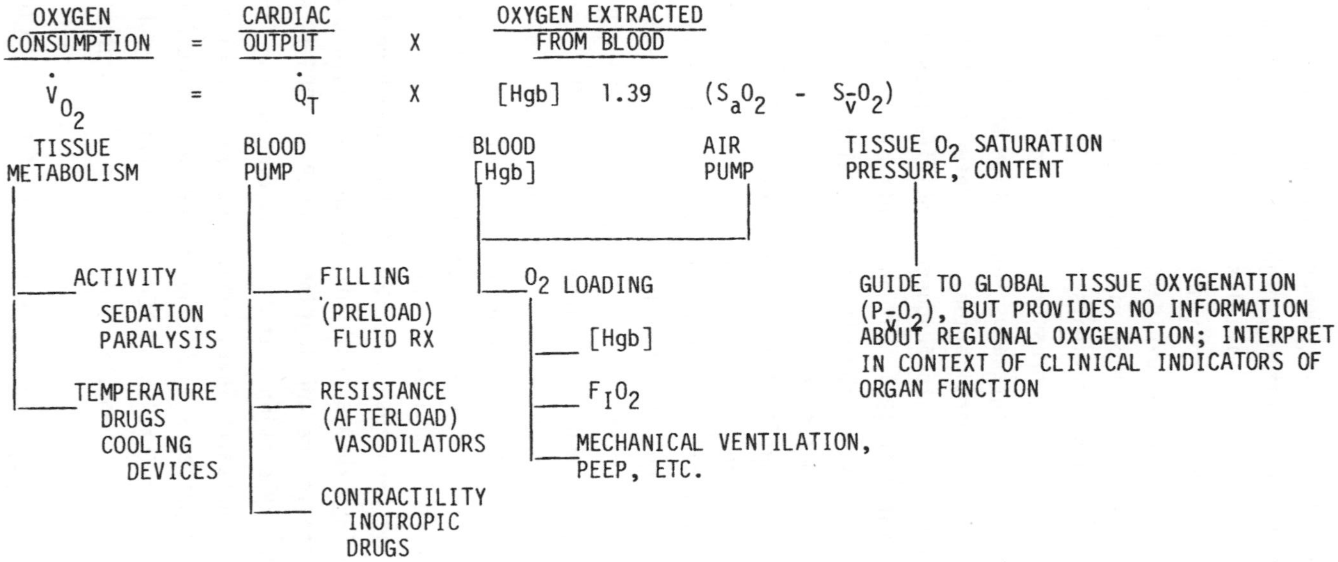

$$\frac{\text{OXYGEN}}{\text{CONSUMPTION}} = \frac{\text{CARDIAC}}{\text{OUTPUT}} \times \text{OXYGEN EXTRACTED FROM BLOOD}$$

$$\dot{V}_{O_2} = \dot{Q}_T \times 1.39 \; [\text{Hgb}] \; (S_aO_2 - S_{\bar{v}}O_2)$$

TISSUE METABOLISM — BLOOD PUMP — BLOOD [Hgb] — AIR PUMP — TISSUE O_2 SATURATION PRESSURE, CONTENT

ACTIVITY
SEDATION
PARALYSIS

FILLING
(PRELOAD)
FLUID RX

O_2 LOADING — [Hgb]

TEMPERATURE
DRUGS
COOLING
DEVICES

RESISTANCE
(AFTERLOAD)
VASODILATORS

F_IO_2

CONTRACTILITY
INOTROPIC
DRUGS

MECHANICAL VENTILATION, PEEP, ETC.

GUIDE TO GLOBAL TISSUE OXYGENATION ($P_{\bar{v}}O_2$), BUT PROVIDES NO INFORMATION ABOUT REGIONAL OXYGENATION; INTERPRET IN CONTEXT OF CLINICAL INDICATORS OF ORGAN FUNCTION

* MODIFIED FROM REFERENCE 27.

1. <u>Oxygen.</u> Because of "refractory hypoxemia" (Table 1) due to lung units that act as intrapulmonary shunts, or have very low ventilation-to-perfusion ratios, high fractions of inspired oxygen (FIO_2) are required in the initial support of the patient.

2. <u>Positive Pressure Ventilation.</u> In practice, this involves the application of positive end expiratory pressure (PEEP) and usually requires mechanical ventilation via an indwelling endotracheal tube, although carefully-chosen patients can occasionally be managed by continuous positive airway pressure delivered by mask. Ventilatory patterns that include spontaneous ventilation by the patient (such as intermittent mandatory ventilation) are preferred, but have not been proven to be superior. High frequency positive pressure ventilation has generated much interest (29), but an insufficient number of patients with ARDS have been supported with this modality to determine if it offers clear advantages over conventional ventilatory patterns.

The physiologic effects and complications of PEEP have been reviewed (29-31). There is no current evidence that PEEP reverses cellular or biochemical aspects of the alveolar capillary lung injury in ARDS, since it does not decrease lung water (30-32) and does not hasten the resolution of experimental lung injury (33). PEEP usually does improve gas exchange and allows lowering of the FIO_2, and thus presumably lessens the chance of O_2 toxicity (9). Since it is a supportive rather than a therapeutic modality, and has potentially-lethal side effects that can affect a variety of organ systems (30-32), its use must be individualized. Several regimens for the application of PEEP in ARDS have been advocated (29-30) but none have been shown to be superior or to favorably affect outcome in controlled trials. A rational approach to the application of PEEP in ARDS is aimed at adequate tissue oxygenation with the reduction of the FIO_2 to an arbitrarily-chosen "safe" level (34). The exact level of inspired O_2 that is safe for patients with lung injury has not been established. The prophylactic application of PEEP to patients at risk for ARDS, but who have not yet developed the syndrome, does not prevent its development (9,34,42).

3. <u>Control of Vascular Hydrostatic Pressure and Fluid Management.</u> In the acute phase of ARDS, when increased pulmonary

capillary permeability is a constant feature, fluid management is aimed at achieving the lowest possible pulmonary capillary hydrostatic pressure in order to minimize the transfer of fluid into the lung parenchyma. The second principle is that this must be accomplished while maintaining cardiac filling pressures that are adequate to support the cardiac output and to maintain blood flow, and oxygen delivery, to critical organs. Attainment of this goal may be complicated by the effects of positive pressure ventilation on cardiac output (29,31) and by underlying cardiovascular alterations (17).

The application of these principles of fluid management has not been shown to improve the outcome of ARDS in controlled studies, but the approach is physiologically sound (12,13,21) and is supported by careful studies with experimental animals (35). It should be emphasized that this approach is aimed at minimizing the accumulation of lung edema, but is not known to influence the cellular dysfunction that is the cause of the increased permeability, and therefore may be unlikely to directly influence the course of lung injury. In individual patients, the approach to fluid management may require various combinations of volume loading, ionotropic and vasoactive agents, and/or diuretics. A number of regimens, using various vasoactive agents and clinical endpoints, have been described (34-38) but none have been shown in controlled fashion to favorably affect the course of human ARDS. It is likely that this aspect of the management will continue to require individualization, in view of the variation in cardiovascular function in patients with ARDS (17).

The choice of intravascular fluid used for resuscitation and volume manipulation in patients with ARDS has been the topic of much debate. The administration of colloid-containing fluids has been advocated. However, the ability of colloid-containing fluids to favorably affect lung edema, in the face of increased permeability of the lung microvessels to protein as well as water, has no physiologic basis. The lack of utility of albumin solutions in experimental alveolar capillary injury has been documented (35,39). Current evidence supports the use of blood (if needed to provide red blood cells for their O_2 carrying capacity) and/or crystalloid fluids, unless colloid-containing fluids are required for other purposes.

4. <u>Cardiovascular Monitoring and Management.</u> Arterial cannulation
is commonly done to facilitate arterial blood gas measurement and to
monitor systemic blood pressure. Pulmonary artery catheterization is
commonly utilized in the management of ARDS, but it has not been shown
to favorably affect the course of the syndrome. We currently believe
that pulmonary artery catheterization is useful in many patients with
ARDS for monitoring during the application of PEEP and because of the
frequency with which multifactorial cardiovascular dysfunction is found
(17). The major indications for this invasive procedure are: A)
measurement of the pulmonary capillary wedge pressure, as an index of
lung capillary hydrostatic pressure, to document increased pulmonary
capillary permeability (Table 1); it must be kept in mind, however, that
mean left atrial pressure, as indicated by the wedge pressure, is an
imprecise measure of pulmonary capillary hydrostatic pressure (13); B)
monitoring of wedge pressure and cardiac output during fluid
manipulation, the administration of vasoactive agents to decrease lung
microvascular pressure (35-37), and the application of PEEP; C)
monitoring during the manipulation of cardiac output to improve O_2
delivery (Figure 1), or during attempts to reduce pulmonary artery
pressure and right ventricular afterload (40); D) monitoring mixed
venous oxygen pressure and saturation (Figure 1).

5. <u>Empiric Use of Glucocorticoids.</u> The administration of
pharmacologic doses of glucocorticoids was advocated for the treatment
of ARDS shortly after the original descriptions of the syndrome (28).
Glucocorticoids, in large doses, continue to be given by many physicians
for the prophylaxis of ARDS and for treatment of the established
syndrome. Currently there is no conclusive evidence, however, that
these drugs alter the course of established ARDS. An uncontrolled study
indicated improvement in alveolar capillary permeability in patients
with sepsis who were given pharmacologic doses of glucocorticoids (44),
although it is not clear from this report if the patients had all
criteria for ARDS (Table 1) and at what point in the natural history of
the syndrome they were studied. The efficacy of glucocorticoids in the
prophylaxis of ARDS is yet to be proven (41,56). Two multicenter trials
that will address this question are in progress.

Prognosis of Adult Respiratory Distress Syndrome: In several recent
reports, the mortality of patients with ARDS was 50-80%
(7,8,17,18,45). This is no lower than that originally reported for ARDS
(1,28), in spite of the evolution of the practice of intensive care and
the application of new technology (43) in the 16 year interval between
the description of ARDS and the present. This suggests that, although
critical evaluation and improvement of supportive measures (modalities
of mechanical ventilation, management of edema, cardiopulmonary
monitoring, etc.) is important, improvement in survival in ARDS may not
occur until a fundamental understanding of the pathophysiology of the
syndrome is available.

Mechanisms of Lung Injury in ARDS: The failure of "state-of-the-art"
supportive measures to favorably influence mortality in ARDS has
stimulated investigations of the cellular and biochemical mechanisms
involved in diffuse alveolar capillary injury. One line of
investigation has been aimed at finding markers of pulmonary endothelial
injury, such as alterations in plasma angiotensin converting enzyme
levels (47) or circulating Factor VIII antigen (48). Such a marker
might provide an index that could be followed during the evolution of
the syndrome, clarifying its natural history. A second approach has
involved studies of mechanisms that may initiate or amplify alveolar
capillary injury (2,6,9,18,49). Table 2 summarizes some of the
mechanisms currently under investigation in experimental models of lung
cell injury, and which have been examined in studies of patients with
ARDS (15,18,47-54). A third line of investigation involves an attempt
to clarify the factors that regulate lung repair after diffuse alveolar
capillary injury (9,49). The intent of these investigations is to
provide knowledge of the basic cellular and biochemical mechanisms that
are active in lung injury and repair in ARDS, so that strategies for
prevention and therapy, rather than simply support of the patient after
the syndrome develops, can be defined. In some cases experimental
observations have suggested the possibility of new therapeutic
approaches (9,56) that are now undergoing experimental evaluation
(57,58).

Table 2

PROPOSED MECHANISMS OF ALVEOLAR CAPILLARY INJURY IN ARDS

1. Injury to Alveolar Lining Cells (Type I & Type II Pneumocytes)
   A. Direct injury (gastric acid, O_2 and O_2 metabolites, viral infection, etc)
   B. Release of proteases (esp. elastase) by neutrophils
   C. Inactivation of antiprotease activity by oxidants generated by inflammatory cells or lung parenchymal cells
2. Injury to Endothelial Cells
   A. Direct injury (O_2 and O_2 metabolites)
   B. Cellular Mediators
      1. Polymorphonuclear leukocytes
      2. Platelets
   C. Humoral Mediators
      1. Complement fragments and other chemotactic factors
      2. Arachidonic acid metabolites (thromboxane A_2, leukotrienes, others)
      3. Platelet-activating factor (1-alkyl-2-acetyl-sn-glycero-3-phosphocholine)
      4. Products of the coagulation cascade: fibrin, fibrin degradation products, thrombin, others
      5. Bradykinin, histamine, others

Acknowledgement: This work was supported in part by Public Health Service Clinical Investigator Award No. HL-00696 from the National Heart, Lung and Blood Institute. The author thanks Jerri Duncan-Goff for her expert preparation of the manuscript.

REFERENCES
1. Ashbaugh DG et al. Acute respiratory distress in adults. Lancet 2:319, 1967.
2. Murray JF. Conference report: Mechanisms of acute respiratory failure. Am Rev Resp Dis 115:1071, 1977.
3. Petty TH. Adult respiratory distress syndrome. Sem Resp Med 2:99, 1981.
4. Petty TL. Adult respiratory distress syndrome: Definition and historical perspective. Clin Chest Med 3:3, 1982.
5. Hopewell PC, Murray JF. The adult respiratory distress syndrome. Ann Rev Med 27:343, 1976.

6. Bone RC, editor. The adult respiratory distress syndrome. Clin Chest Med 3:1-215, 1982.
7. Fowler AA et al. Adult respiratory distress syndrome: Risk with common predispositions. Ann Int Med 98:593, 1983.
8. Pepe PE et al. Clinical predictors of the adult respiratory distress syndrome. Am J Surg 144:124, 1982.
9. Rinaldo JE, Rogers RM. Adult respiratory distress syndrome. Changing concepts of lung injury and repair. N Eng J Med 206:900, 1982.
10. Bachofen M, Weibel ER. Structural alterations of lung parenchyma in the adult respiratory distress syndrome. Clin Chest Med 3:35, 1982.
11. Anderson RR et al. Documentation of pulmonary capillary permeability in the adult respiratory distress syndrome accompanying human sepsis. Am Rev Resp Dis 119:869, 1979.
12. Albert RK. Factors affecting transvascular fluid and protein movement in pulmonary edema and ARDS. Sem Resp Med 2:102, 1981.
13. Staub NC. The pathogenesis of pulmonary edema. Prog Cardiovasc Dis 23:53, 1980.
14. Greene R et al. Early bedside detection of pulmonary vascular occlusion during acute respiratory failure. Am Rev Resp Dis 124:593, 1981.
15. Elliott CG et al. Granulocyte aggregation in adult respiratory distress syndrome (ARDS): Serial histologic and physiologic observations. Am J Med Sci: In Press, September, 1984.
16. Zapol WM, Snider MT. Pulmonary hypertension in severe acute respiratory failure. N Eng J Med 296:476, 1977.
17. Zimmerman GA et al. Cardiovascular alterations in the adult respiratory distress syndrome. Am J Med 73:25, 1982.
18. Zimmerman GA et al. Functional and metabolic activity of granulocytes from patients with adult respiratory distress syndrome: evidence for activated neutrophils in the pulmonary circulation. Am Rev Resp Dis 127:290, 1983.
19. Snow RL et al. Pulmonary vascular remodeling in adult respiratory distress syndrome. Am Rev Resp Dis 126:887, 1982.
20. Staub NC. Pulmonary edema. Physiologic approaches to management. Chest 74: 559, 1978.
21. Brigham K et al. Increased sheep lung vascular permeability caused by E. Coli endotoxin. Circ Res 45:292, 1979.
22. Hallman M et al. Evidence of lung surfactant abnormality in respiratory failure. J Clin Invest 70:673, 1982.
23. Pingleton SK. Complications associated with the adult respiratory distress syndrome. Clin Chest Med 3:143, 1982.
24. Bell RC et al. Multiple organ system failure and infection in adult respiratory distress syndrome. Ann Int Med 99:293, 1983.
25. Hudson LD. Causes of the adult respiratory distress syndrome: Clinical recognition. Clin Chest Med 3:195, 1982.
26. Wiedmann HP et al. Cardiovascular-pulmonary monitoring in the intensive care unit. Chest 85:537, 1984.
27. Morris AH. Clinical application of the Fick Equation. Pulmonary Fellow's Handbook, Intermountain Respiratory Intensive Care Unit, LDS Hospital, Salt Lake City, Utah, 1976.
28. Petty TL, Ashbaugh DG. The adult respiratory distress syndrome. Clinical features, factors influencing prognosis, and principles of management. Chest 60:233, 1971.

156

29. Gong H. Positive-pressure ventilation in the adult respiratory distress syndrome. Clin Chest Med 3:69, 1982.
30. Weisman IM et al. Positive end-expiratory pressure in adult respiratory failure. N Eng J Med 307:1381, 1982.
31. Tyler DC. Positive end expiratory pressure: A review. Crit Care Med 11:300, 1983.
32. Rizk NW, Murray J. PEEP and pulmonary edema. Am J Med 72:381, 1982.
33. Luce J et al. The effects of expiratory positive airway pressure on the resolution of oleic acid-induced lung injury in dogs. Am Rev Resp Dis 125:716, 1982.
34. Hudson LD. Adult respiratory distress syndrome. In RM Cherniack (editor), Current Therapy of Respiratory Disease 1984-1985. BC Decker, Inc, Philadelphia, 1984, PP 284.
35. Prewitt RM et al. Treatment of acute low pressure pulmonary edema in dogs. Relative effects of hydrostatic and oncotic pressure, nitroprusside, and positive end expiratory pressure. J Clin Invest 67:409, 1981.
36. Wood LDH, Prewitt RM. Cardiovascular management in acute hypoxemic respiratory failure. Am J Card 47:963, 1981.
37. Ghingnone M et al. Effects of hydralazine on cardiopulmonary function in canine low-pressure pulmonary edema. Anesthesiol 59:187, 1983.
38. Matamis D et al. Redistribution of pulmonary blood flow induced by positive end expiratory pressure and dopamine infusion in acute respiratory failure. Am Rev Resp Dis 129:39, 1984.
39. Nanjo S et al. Concentrated albumin does not affect lung edema formation after acid instillation in the dog. Am Rev Resp Dis 126:884, 1983.
40. Prewitt RM, Ghingnone M. Treatment of right ventricular dysfunction in acute respiratory failure. Crit Care Med 11:346, 1983.
41. Nicholson DP. Glucocorticoids in the treatment of shock and the adult respiratory distress syndrome. Clin Chest Med 3:121, 1982.
42. Pepe PE et al. Early application of PEEP in patients at risk for ARDS. Am Rev Resp Dis 127:97A, 1983.
43. Pontoppidan H et al. Respiratory intensive care. Anesthesiol 47:96, 1977.
44. Sibbald WJ et al. Alveolar-capillary permeability in human septic ARDS. Effect of high-dose corticosteroid therapy. Chest 79:133, 1981.
45. Fein AM et al. The risk factors, incidence, and prognosis of ARDS following septicemia. Chest 83:40, 1983.
46. Clemmer TP, Orme JF. Nutritional support in the adult respiratory distress syndrome. Clin Chest Med 3:101, 1982.
47. Fourrier F et al. Angiotensin converting enzyme in human adult respiratory distress syndrome. Chest 83:593, 1983.
48. Carvalho A et al. Altered factor VIII in acute respiratory failure. N Eng J Med 307:1113, 1982.
49. Repine JE (editor). Lung defense, injury and repair. Chest 83:(Supplement):1 S-103 S, 1983.
50. Hammerschmidt DE et al. Association of complement activation and elevated plasma-C5a with adult respiratory distress syndrome. Pathophysiologic relevance and possible prognostic value. Lancet 1:947, 1980.

51. Zimmerman GA et al. Granulocyte adherence in pulmonary and systemic arterial blood samples from patients with adult respiratory distress syndrome. Am Rev Resp Dis 129:798, 1984.
52. Schneider RC et al. Platelet consumption and sequestration in severe acute respiratory failure. Am Rev Resp Dis 122:445, 1980.
53. Haynes JB et al. Elevated fibrinogen degradation products in the adult respiratory distress syndrome. Am Rev Resp Dis 122:841, 1980.
54. Cochran CG et al. The presence of neutrophil elastase and evidence of oxidation activity in bronchoalveolar lavage fluid of patients with adult respiratory distress syndrome. Am Rev Resp Dis 127:S25-S27, 1983.
55. Chand N, Altura BM. Acetylcholine and bradykinin relax intrapulmonary arteries by acting on endothelial cells: Role in lung vascular diseases. Science 213:1376, 1981.
56. Sprung CL et al. Effects of corticosteroids on the incidence of the adult respiratory distress syndrome (ARDS) in patients with septic shock: A prospective study. Am Rev Resp Dis 129:A102, 1984.
57. Ogletree ML, Brigham KL. PGE_1 reduces lung transvascular filtration during endotoxin-induced high permeability in sheep. Clin Res 27:402A, 1979.
58. Appel PL, Shoemaker WC. Effect of prostaglandin (E_1) on hemodynamic and oxygen transport in ARDS. Crit Care Med 11:242, 1983.
59. Zapol WM et al. L-3,4-dehydroproline suppression of fibrosis in ARDS: Early clinical results. Am Rev Resp Dis 1984:129, A102.

BASIC UNDERSTANDING OF INTRAPULMONARY PERCUSSIVE VENTILATION
IPV

FORREST M. BIRD, M.D., PH.D., SC.D.

Bird Intrapulmonary Percussive Ventilation is a form of physical therapy, administered to the pulmonary airways by a pneumatic (air) device called a Percussionator.

The patient breathes through a mouthpiece that delivers high flow mini-bursts of air into the lungs at rates of over two hundred times each minute.

During the percussive bursts of air into the lungs, a continued pressure wedge is maintained, while a high velocity flow opens airways and enhances intrabronchial secretion mobilization.

A specific medication called racemic epinephrine in a 2.25% aqueous concentration (6 drops) is diluted with 20cc of water and aerosolized into the lungs by a special mist generator.

The aerosol mist is delivered throughout the lungs during therapeutic percussion by the intrapulmonary Percussionator[TM]. Aerosol misting within the lungs reduces the adhesive and cohesive forces of retained airway secretions, decreases swelling within the walls of the pulmonary airways and relaxes potential spasm of the terminal bronchioles (small airways) of the lungs.

160

Each percussive interval is programmed by the patient.
Normally, the patient holds the thumb button depressed for a
five to ten second interval. While the thumb button is held
depressed, the lungs are shaken up, mixing intrapulmonary
oxygen, carbon dioxide and nitrogen with a medicated mist.
At the end of the percussive interval, the thumb button is
released, allowing exhalation of the well mixed
intrapulmonary gases from the lungs.

After each exhalation, the percussive interval starts anew,
refilling the lungs with fresh moist medicated respiratory
gases. The cyclical intrapulmonary exchange of well mixed
respiratory gases serves to flush out carbon dioxide and
renew oxygen.

Whenever there is a desire to cough or expectorate, the
thumb button is released until the coughing episode is
completed or secretions are raised and cleared. A routine
IPV therapy period lasts approximately twenty minutes.

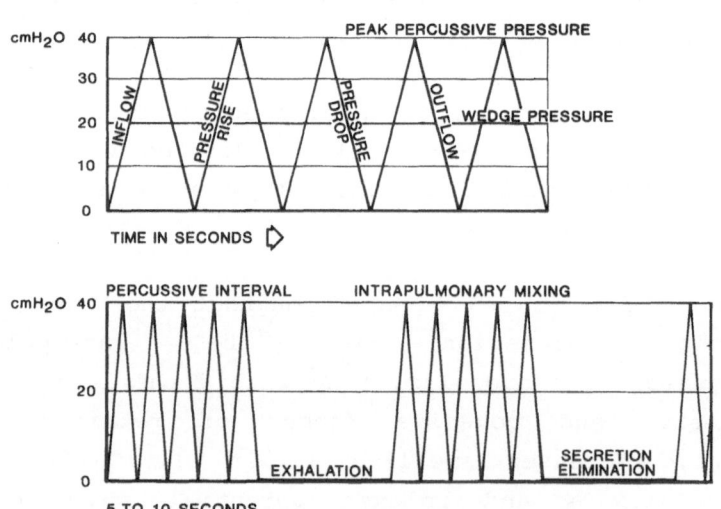

Theoretical pressure tracings and intervals.

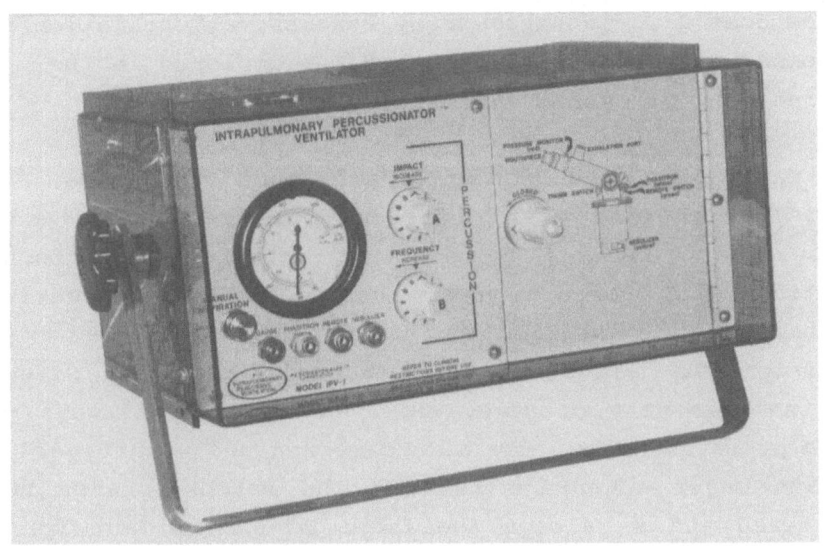

IPV-1 Percussionator for administering Bird
Intrapulmonary Percussive Ventilation.

Basic percussive programming is controlled by adjustments to
two knobs. The IMPACT control knob is usually set at the
12:00 index arrow. Rotation (against the clock) increases
impact flow time, creating the delivery of larger air
bursts. The FREQUENCY control knob is also normally set at
12:00 index arrow. Rotation (against the clock) increases
the number of impacts (air bursts) each minute. The airway
manometer dial measures the average (mean) intrapulmonary
wedge pressure.

Normally, a 30 psi operating pressure is an optimal starting
point. Increasing operational pressures from 30 toward 50
psig increases flow velocity during impact. Therefore, the
force of impact can be increased by increasing the velocity
of flow. The intrapulmonary wedge pressure is increased by
increasing frequency of impact pulses.

How does Bird Intrapulmonary Percussive Ventilation
compare to chest physiotherapy, as employed in the
treatment of cystic fibrosis, etc?

Very favorably, the concepts are much the same. The
percussive shock waves of both methods are transmitted to
the pulmonary airways to mobilize retained endobronchial
secretions. A Percussionator could be very effectively
programmed by a skilled pulmonary physiotherapist. The·
Percussionator delivering the percussive impulses directly
into the pulmonary airways, while holding the airways open
with a pressure wedge, may have a mechanical advantage. One
definite major advantage is that the Percussionator never
gets tired and is always available to the patient for the
self-administration of intrapulmonary percussion at his or
her convenience.

When IPV therapy is employed for the long term
management of obstructive pulmonary diseases, what might
be expected in terms of controlling the basic diseases?

With the primary causes of chronic obstructive
cardiopulmonary diseases obscure, there is no one defining
treatment directed toward the cause. Therefore, all
treatment has been primarily directed at amelioration of
symptoms with minimal effect upon the reduction of the
insidious progression of the disease. While lack of
clinical knowledge may limit cause and effect relationships,
in terms of optimal clinical efficacy, a logical compromise
must be carefully rationalized.

When chronic obstructive pulmonary disease accelerators are studied, the most direct known accelerator is the chronic obstruction of the pulmonary airways. If pulmonary emphysema is considered, in part, an eschemic (blood supply) disease, a potentially effective clinical management protocol might be directed at a reduction of blood supply embarrassment. Therefore, the earlier such a clinical regime is enacted after initial diagnosis, the greater the long term effectivity.

Mucosal and submucosal edema of the pulmonary airways most likely serves to reduce both systemic and pulmonary blood flow, secondary to vesicular compression of unknown degree.

The end result of long term encroachment upon the systemic and pulmonary circulations of the lung is predictable.

The asthmatic patient, with his or her obstructive pulmonary disease component, does not appear to have the same tendency to develop pulmonary emphysema that is associated with chronic bronchitis. Is this explained because the asthmatic has considerable remission and is devoid of the long term unrelenting airway obstruction associated with chronic bronchitis?

With this further rationalization of factors and accelerators associated with chronic obstructive pulmonary diseases, the logic for Bird conceived Intrapulmonary Percussive Ventilation can be explored.

Treatment of the cause of chronic obstructive pulmonary disease is quite impossible because the absolute factors of the diseases remain unknown; therefore, secondary therapeutic means must be advanced. These measures must therefore be primarily directed toward the limitation of known accelerators of the disease process with associated amelioration of symptoms.

It was upon this basis that Bird conceived the therapeutic
protocol defined as IPV.

During the percussive interval, IPV maintains an
intrapulmonary wedge pressure serving to stabilize airway
patency (size). With the maintenance of a mean (average)
wedge pressure (mechanical obturator), a repetitive
percussive pressure change (through the wedge pressure)
serves as a pneumatic air hammer to open obstructed
pulmonary airways by breaching retained endobronchial
secretions.

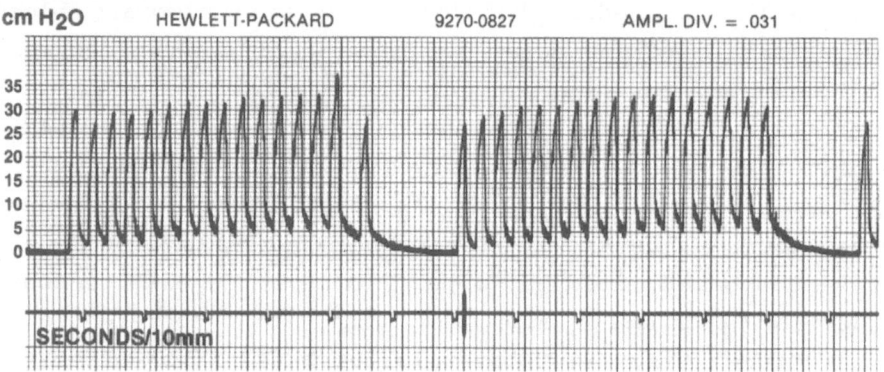

An actual IPV pressure wave form measured at the proximal
physiological airway.

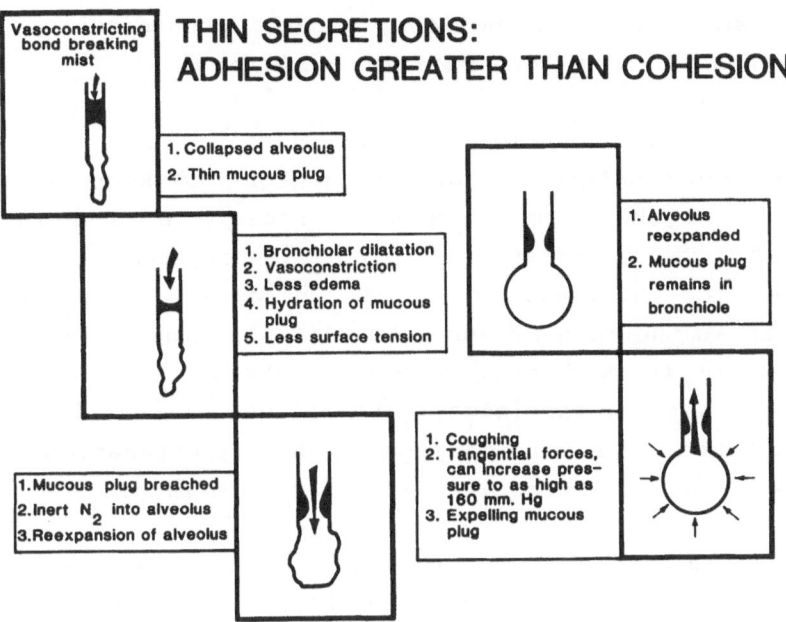

The possible oversimplified mobilization of thin secretions.

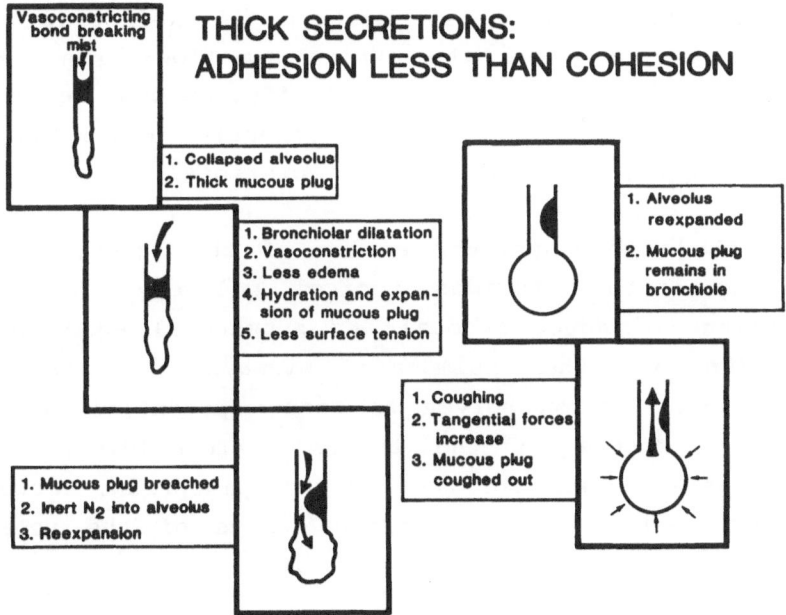

Possible oversimplified mobilization of thick secretions.

After airway breaching and the delivery of an air distal to the endobronchial obstructions, a basic mechanical means of endobronchial secretion mobilization begins.

Concomitant to mechanical airway dilation, an aerosolized topical vasoconstrictor, bronchodilator and secretion bond breaker, in the form of aqueous racemic epinephrine, is delivered in a therapeutic mist. During the percussive therapeutic interval, forceful pulsatile intrabronchial impulses at the rate of about 200-500 per minute, serve most effectively to mechanically mix (shake up) intrapulmonary gases and aerosol particles. The diffuse bilateral delivery and exchange of respiratory gases during percussion serves to provide a more effective blood gas interface.

After intrapulmonary gas mixing during the five to ten second percussive interval, the proximal airway pressures are dropped to ambient. With an effective volume of inspiratory gases in the peripheral pulmonary structures, under positive pressures, a major flow gradient to ambient from the distal pulmonary airways is affected. This substantially increases the expiratory flow volume rate. The greater the expiratory flow velocity, as compared to the inspiratory flow rates, the more effective the mechanical removal of retained endobronchial secretions.

Through the vasoconstrictor action of the agent, the IPV aerosol generator provides topical delivery of racemic epinephrine to reduce mucosal and submucosal edema within the walls of the pulmonary airways. A secondary bronchodilator action serves to reduce potential spasm of the smooth muscle of the terminal bronchioles. Water employed as a diluent for the racemic epinephrine serves to lower both adhesive and cohesive forces of the retained endobronchial secretions, thus serving as a bond breaking vehicle.

Therefore, IPV serves as a medium to mechanically and chemically mobilize endobronchial secretions. This includes:

1. Maintaining and percussing the pulmonary airways.
2. Delivering a topical aerosolized vasoconstrictor, bronchodilator and bond breaker to reduce endobronchial congestion.
3. Enhancing an expiratory flow velocity advancing the cephalad mobilization of retained endobronchial secretions.

IPV appears to be a most effective means of routinely reducing airway congestion, temporarily reversing the three components of airway obstruction. The effective period of increased diffuse airway caliber varies with patient and activity. Generally, three daily IPV treatments four hours apart serve to maintain a substantial pulmonary airway with an associated decrease in alveolar hyperinflation (FRC).

By partially breaking the chronic pulmonary airway obstruction and associated alveolar hyperinflation for prolonged periods on a routine basis, the critical threshold for effective systemic and pulmonary blood flow may be maintained, with an associated reduction in the ischemic deterioration of the peripheral pulmonary structures. Therefore, IPV therapy may well be the most effective clinical protocol directed toward the maximum mobilization of pulmonary airway obstruction and provide long term prophylactic management.

If emphysema is an ischemic pulmonary disease, secondary to a reduction in systemic peripheral perfusion within the pulmonary structures, any therapeutic protocol that would serve to increase perfusion might well serve to reduce the insidious progression in proportion to the maintenance of increased blood flow.

One factor that would be hard to deny is that by increasing peripheral air exchange, the partial pressures of oxygen in the peripheral pulmonary structures will be increased. As peripheral oxygen tensions are increased, a pulmonary capillary dilation would be expected, which in turn would reduce the pulmonary vascular resistance between the right and left heart. This would provide for a lower pulmonary artery pressure serving to decrease the work of the right heart. Therefore, existing right heart strain (cor pulmonale) would be ameliorated.

This general treatise has been based, in part, upon a five year study of IPV in patients of all ages with all forms of cardiopulmonary diseases. While certain clinical evidence remains subjective, objectivity is increasing as the size of the reporting patient population is rapidly expanding.

There are several other important considerations associated with IPV that remain to be confirmed or denied. They are:
1. Does the intrapulmonary percussion have sufficient amplitude to increase pulmonary lymph flow? If this is the case, does the reduction in lung water enhance the diffusive activity across the alveolar capillary membranes? This could be a major contribution.
2. Could the percussive pulse create a vesicular peristalsis, creating a forward enhancement of systemic and pulmonary flow? This could produce a secondary influence in the maintenance of a viable peripheral circulation within the lungs.
3. Finally, a number of initial control patients treated with uninterrupted IPV for over four years continue to subjectively improve. This controlled patient population represents chronic patients maintained under excellent medical supervision for at least ten years before commencing IPV therapy.

Can this improvement be explained by the increased efficacy in the control over endobronchial secretion only? Possibly, however, more likely an enhancement to perfusive activity, resultant from or associated with the protocol, may remain to be evidenced.

BASIC UNDERSTANDING OF VOLUMETRIC DIFFUSIVE RESPIRATION
VDR

FORREST M. BIRD, M.D., PH.D., SC.D.

The Bird VDR concepts were theoretically advanced as a means
of providing for a ventilatory device that would allow
control over intrabronchial diffusion as well as convection.
As prototype device became available, the concept was
advanced to a universal ventilatory system. At this point
in time, one mechanical device can be programmed to
accommodate a multiplicity of diffusive and convective wave
forms. The IPV/VDR concepts appear to function equally well
in all age groups with compound cardiopulmonary
pathophysiology.

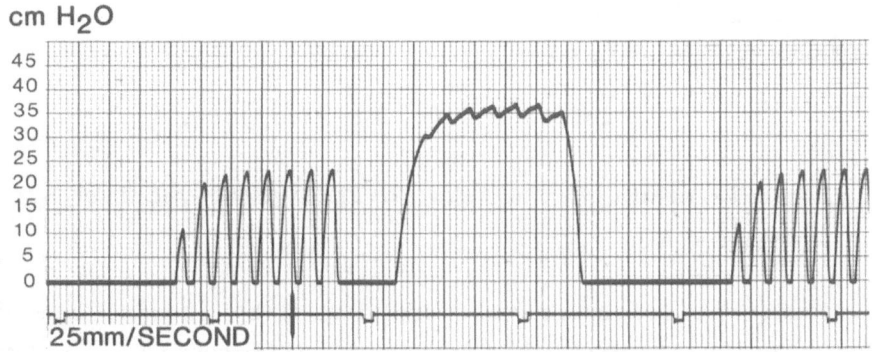

Typical Bird conceived Volumetric Diffusive Respiration
(VDR) wave form.

The basic Bird VDR wave form breaks down into several
segments:

A. Percussive/diffusive segment, predominatly
    influencing PaO_2.

B. Diffusive/convective transition segment,
    predominatly influencing $PaCO_2$.

C. Convective tidal delivery segment, predominantly
    influencing $PaCO_2$.

D. Post tidal baseline pause segment, influences
    cardiac output by providing time for
    systemic/pulmonary volume equilibration with a
    predominant influence on $PaCO_2$.

E. Static CPAP/PEEP baseline elevation segment,
    primarily influences right to left shunting with a
    predominant effect upon PaO_2.

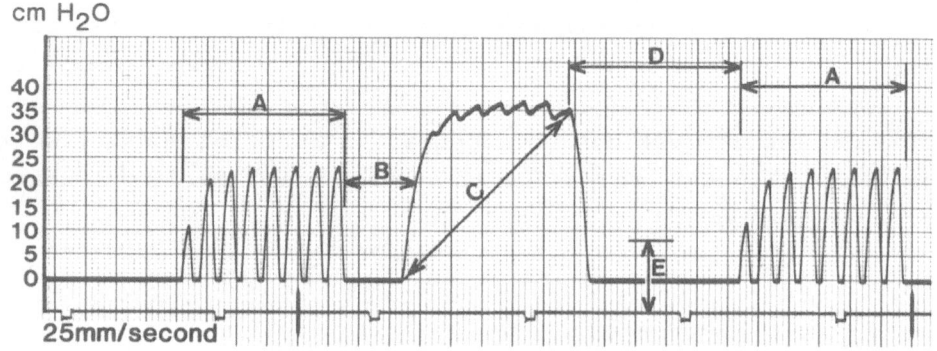

Basic VDR wave form segments.

What is meant by the term "diffusive/convective"
ventilation?

Diffusion is molecular movement caused by thermal agitation
and regional partial pressure differentials. During
spontaneous respiration, approximately 15% of the total lung
volume is tidally exchanged with the intrapulmonary blood
gas interface dependent upon a major diffusive action.
Within the pulmonary structures, the limit of thermal

agitation is about 37° C. Additional diffusive action would be secondary to a turbulent (mechanically induced) high velocity inflow producing an intrapulmonary mechanical mixing. Intrapulmonary mechanical mixing may produce sufficient additional molecular collision to increase frictional heating of the molecular complex. Increasing molecular velocity would thus increase intrapulmonary diffusion. Then a therapeutic FIO_2 prevails, the additional diffusive activity within the pulmonary structures may serve to reflect upon PaO_2.

Within limits, intrapulmonary mechanical mixing can be increased by increasing the velocity and frequency of intrapulmonary stroke volume delivery. Therefore, intrapulmonary diffusion may be increased by the mechanical delivery of higher frequency pulsed stroke volumes into the pulmonary structures.

Convection/conduction, as traditionally employed in referring to the mass molecular tidal flow of respiratory gases in and out of the pulmonary structures, is not totally correct, but is generally accepted. Therefore, a tidal exchange may be understood as a volume of respiratory gas that exceeds the anatomical dead space as opposed to a volume that is less than the anatomical dead space which is referred to as a stroke volume.

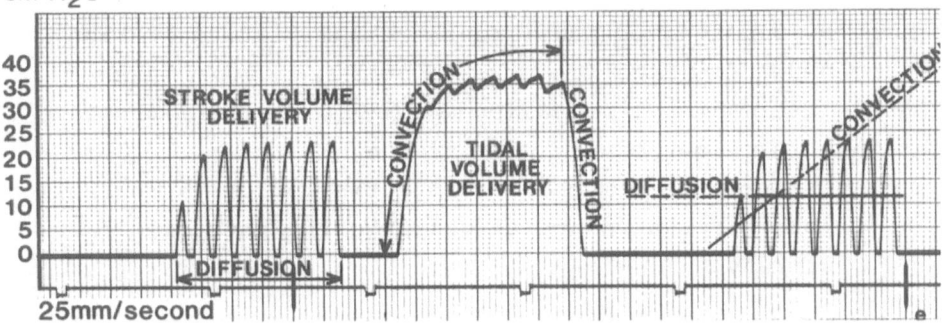

Stroke versus tidal volume with definition of commanding diffusive and convective components.

174

What is a Bird conceived phasitron and what functions does it provide?

The Bird conceived phasitron is a flow converter/synchronization device. Essentially, the square wave pulsed flow generated by the Percussionator^{TM} is amplified, sined (analogued) and synchronized by the phasitron for physiological delivery.

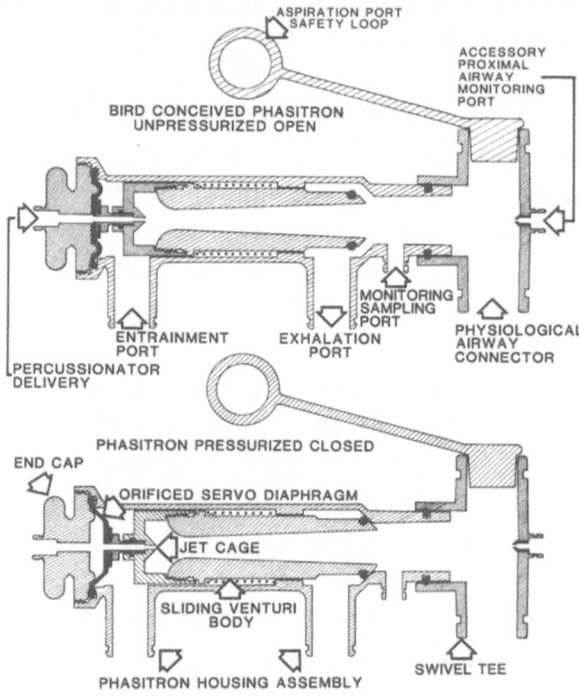

The Bird conceived phasitron in dynamic cross section.

The phasitron might be called a "physiological interface". Cardinal functions of the phasitron are:
1. To provide a method of injecting, under a controlled pressure, a volume of gas into the physiological airway.

2. To amplify the delivery volume by entrainment of a similar gas by as much as five times the jet ejected volume.

3. To conform to changing pulmonary resistances by (automatically) converting flow to pressure and vice versa, within the venturi body of the phasitron. Pneumatic clutching serves to enhance intrapulmonary distribution and to minimize square wave flow dissection potential.

4. To provide for precise synchronization of the inspiratory/expiratory intervals without inertial valving lag as frequency increases. Lag is of major importance in the minimization of functional residual volumes at any given scheduled volume/frequency.

5. To provide for an ambient communication between the physiological and mechanical airways. Ambient venting is a major failsafe factor under all dynamic or static conditions.

6. To provide for monitoring of proximal airway pressures.

7. To provide for flow through, and entrainment of, an aerosolized mist for humidification, bulk water and medication delivery.

8. To prevent the step ladder delivery of intrapulmonary volumes above a scheduled peak proximal airway pressure limit.

9. To provide for the delivery of repetitive stroke volumes through an adjustable mean intrapulmonary pressure wedge.

10. To provide for a competent, durable, easy to maintain ejector/exhalation valve.

Differential ventilation with the VDR Percussionators.

For many years, "jury rigged" appliances have been employed for differential ventilation. Essentially, independent ventilators have been used to synchronously or asychronously administer separate ventilatory protocols. Left and right pulmonary structures have been separated by the insertion of a Carlens type catheter.

Applications for such device have been:

1. Logical manipulation of a single pulmonary structure.
2. A traumatized (shocked) lung with the remaining structure having limited involvement.
3. Abnormal perfusion within intrathoracic pulmonary and systemic circulations.
4. Unilateral lesion, local or diffuse.

Functionally, the basic percussive Volumetric Diffusive Respiration (VDR) devices can be programmed to provide differential ventilation. This is accomplished by utilizing the higher frequency counterpulse to stabilize or ventilate the surgical or traumatized lung.

The Bird VDR pulse and counterpulse are programmed 180° apart. That is, the pulsed (stroke volume) is delivered inspiratorily and the counterpulse is delivered expiratorily. When the counterpulse is connected to the jet of a parallel phasitron, a second stroke volume is delivered counter to the normal inspiratory stroke volume. When the phasitrons are coupled differently to separate lungs, the pulse is employed to ventilate the (control) lung with minimal involvement while the counterpulse ventilates the involved surgical or traumatized structure.

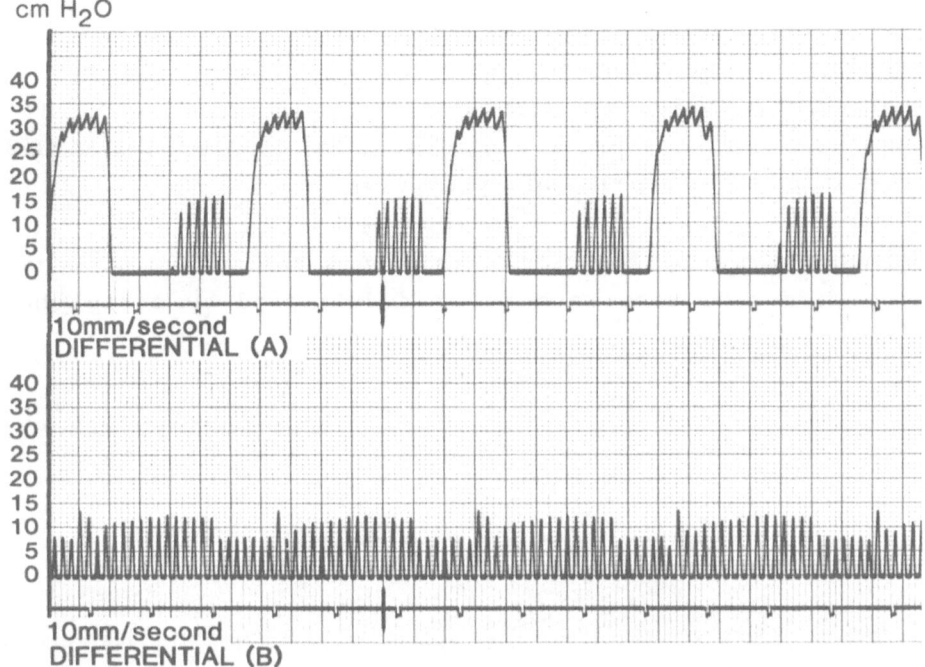

cm H₂O

10mm/second
DIFFERENTIAL (A)

10mm/second
DIFFERENTIAL (B)

Proximal airway pressures at the Carlens interface reveal
the wave forms of Bird VDR differential ventilation.

Accessory enhancement of volumetric diffusive
respiration (VDR) programs.

As clinical VDR research progressed, it has become
increasingly apparent that oscillatory demand CPAP (OD-CPAP)
is more effective under certain circumstances (in the
control over PaO_2 than static PEEP or demand CPAP.

178

In response to clinical demands for greater control over
baseline oscillatory CPAP, Bird created an enhancement
circuit. Essentially, the enhancement circuit allows the
precise programming of an oscillatory CPAP during the
scheduled interruption interval. This may be of
considerable value in maintaining an increased convective
component during a primary diffuse wave form with a minimal
rise in peak intrapulmonary pressures.

Enchancement amplifies the clinician's ability to produce a
true diffusive sine wave as is illustrated by strip chart
tracing.

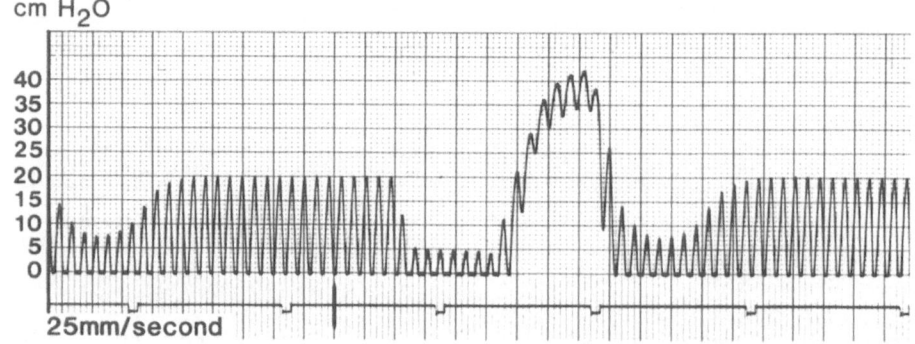

Sine wave diffusive/convective wave form.

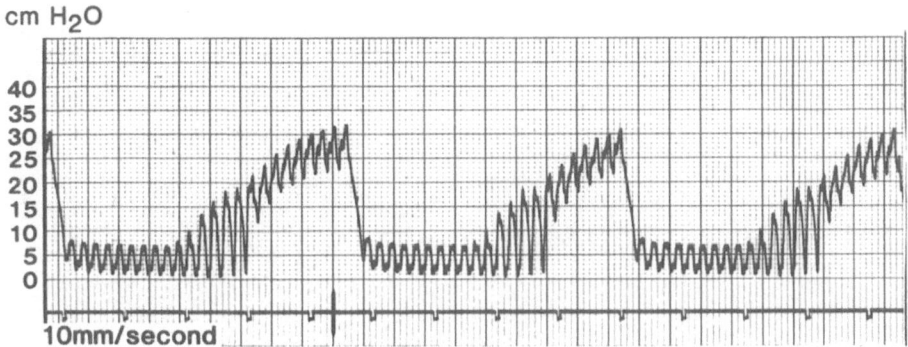

Bird conceived Volumetric Diffusive Respiration (VDR) is a combined program of diffusive and convective techniques.

Bird Volumetric Diffusive Respiration provides a versatile means for long term intensive care ventilatory management. All events can be individually programmed to conform to specific clinical judgment.

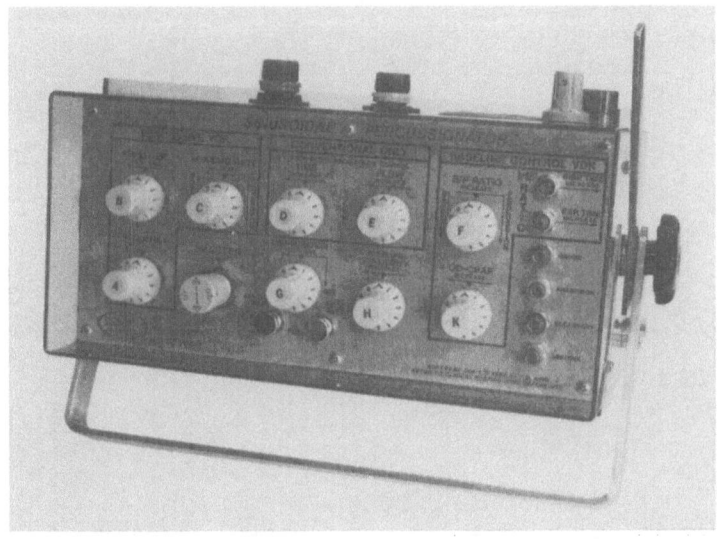

The Percussionaire Sinusoidal Percussionator, Model VDR-1.

THE PATHOPHYSIOLOGY OF CARDIOPULMONARY RESUSCITATION

MARK C. ROGERS, M.D.

Resuscitation is an ancient medical practice which has moved from
folk medicine techniques such as suspending drowning victims upside down to
some semblance of scientific approaches in the last century. Furthermore,
research intensity was increased when anesthetics were developed in the
nineteenth century. Since anesthetics produced not only relief of pain,
but sudden unexpected death, there was a need for the physician to respond.
Large numbers of chloroform deaths stimulated Moritz Schiff,[1] Professor
of Physiology at Florence, to develop cardiac massage and artificial ventilation and demonstrated how to resuscitate dogs. This pioneering work
resulted in the surgical technique of open-chest cardiac compression and
the first recorded human case was reported in a patient undergoing, fitting-
ly enough, chloroform anesthesia.

In the last quarter century, new emphasis in the field of resuscitation
grew when Kouwenhoven[2] popularized closed chest CPR. Now this technique
has been used, not only by physicians, but by emergency medical technicians
and even the public. Major cities have embarked on large scale training
programs for the population. Despite the utility of the technique, it has
become clear in the past few years that the premise on which this closed
chest technique works, by compressing the heart between the sternum and
the vertebral column, is not correct.

This question was raised when Criley[3] reported a patient undergoing
cardiac catheterization who developed simutaneous ventricular fibrillation
and coughing. This combination resulted in sufficient cardiac output such
that the patient remained conscious with an adequate blood pressure despite
the ventricular fibrillation. Clearly the increase in pleural pressure from
the cough was somehow responsible. This observation should have been anticipated, however, since it was related to many scientific observations docu-
menting that pleural pressure changes associated with respiration had the

ability to alter cardiac output. This relationship is the basis for observations relating blood pressure to respiration in pulses paridoxicus, for instance. Regardless, the concept that cardiac output could be maintained during ventricular fibrillation with pleural pressure changes by themselves produced a new theory of cardiopulmonary resuscitation.

Currently, most researchers believe that blood flow during closed-chest CPR results from an increase in intrathoracic pressure produced by chest compression and not from direct cardiac compression. While in small children or thin adults direct cardiac compression can occur, this is not common. During CPR it appears that the elevated pleural pressure increases the pressure in all vascular structures in the chest. This increase in vascular pressure produced by the pleural pressure elevations is transmitted to extrathoracic arteries and results in forward flow of blood during chest compression. This belief was documented by observations in the catheterization laboratory that during CPR the intrathoracic vascular pressures can be transmitted to the extrathoracic arterial bed but not to the venous bed. The reason for this is the presence of competent venous valves at the thoracic inlet. As a result, with chest compression during CPR there is a pressure gradient between arteries and veins outside the thorax which is not related directly to actual cardiac compression but to increased pleural pressure. This is responsible for forward flow of blood. When the chest compression is released, blood flows back into the chest and into the heart.

Many studies[4,5,6] now have clearly documented that in most adult patients cardiac compression does not need to occur in order for there to be aortic blood flow during CPR. Furthermore, techniques which increase intrathoracic pressure during CPR increase both aortic pressure and carotid blood flow. As a result, experiments with alterations in CPR techniques to maximize pleural pressure with simultaneous chest compression and ventilation (SCV) clearly would be logical to maximize cardiac output during CPR. This would maximally raise pleural pressure during CPR. This has been the basis of the concept that simultaneous ventilation and compression (SCV) CPR may produce such higher levels of aortic carotid blood flow that the poor neurologic outcome associated with prolonged CPR can be significantly improved[7,8].

These studies have documented that peripheral blood flow and even carotid arterial blood flow can be improved by simultaneous ventilation and compression (SVC-CPR). Nevertheless, this is not necessarily the desired effect in itself. The reason is that carotid blood flow is not an index of cerebral blood flow and increasing cerebral blood flow is the key to improved neurologic outcome from CPR. To begin, cerebral blood flow may originate from vessels other than the carotid artery such as the vertebral arteries. The most important fact is that the carotid artery blood supplies both the intracranial contents (brain) as well as the extracranial (tongue, cheeks) needs of the head. Furthermore, we know it is theoretically possible to have excellent carotid blood flow. We see this in many patients who are brain dead but who have normal carotid pulses. This is of potential significance since there are data to suggest that the very high levels of pleural pressure seen during CPR may actually result in dramatic increases in intracranial pressure which might limit cerebral blood flow.

In any circumstance, brain blood flow will be related to the difference between mean arterial pressure and mean intracranial pressure and this is referred to as the cerebral perfusion pressure (CPP). With the development of intracranial pressure monitoring, it has been observed that patients on mechanical ventilation who require large amounts of positive end expiratory pressure (PEEP) may have marked elevations in intracranial pressure when the PEEP is applied.[9] As a result, pleural pressure changes associated with CPR may result in dramatic ICP changes. Theoretically, techniques recommended for increasing carotid artery blood flow during CPR (simultaneous ventilation and compression), might actually result in increased carotid and extracranial blood flow but little change in cerebral blood flow itself. Any technique designed to increase blood pressure would be of little value if the intracranial pressure also increases even more than the increase in blood pressure.

This possibility was documented when Rogers et al.[11] first noted in patients monitored with intracranial pressure monitoring devices that there was a direct relationship between chest compression and ICP during CPR. These patients had Swan Ganz catheters, (pulmonary artery pressure, and right atrial pressure) and radial artery pressures in addition to ICP monitors and demonstrated that when the chest was compressed during CPR, there was an increase in intrathoracic pressure and an increase in radial artery pressure. Simultaneously, there was also an increase in pressure. Cerebral perfusion pressure could not increase as a result. Now confirmed, these studies have been extended to animals. There appears to be a direct relationship between the magnitude of intrathoracic pressure rise produced by CPR and the height of the ICP. Clearly, direct measurements of cerebral blood flow are vital for interpretation of any maneuvers designed to alter CPR.

Currently work in our laboratory has been done examining if simultaneous ventilation and compression techniques have the potential of improving cerebral blood flow during CPR. We have been able to document that, in this experimental setting, cerebral blood flow increases with simultaneous ventilation compression CPR.[6] The reason is that the total rise in blood pressure is greater than the total rise in intracranial pressure and the rate of rise in blood pressure is greater than the rise in intracranial pressure. As a result total cerebral perfusion pressure as well as the time available for perfusion to the brain is increased and cerebral blood flow improves.

This work also raises the question of how best to take advantage of the dramatic increase in carotid blood flow seen with SVC-CPR. It is possible to conceive that if extracranial resistance is increased pharmacologically, carotid blood flow would be directed to the brain. Michael[12] has now conducted a series of experiments which document that epinephrine improves cerebral blood flow to the brain, even above pre-arrest values in certain settings, if used with SCV-CPR. This appears to be due to alpha agonist properties and is associated with a normal EGG pattern during nearly one hour of CPR.

Future developments in CPR are likely to be directed as improving the redistribution of carotid blood flow with a wide variety of agents. Foremost among the promising agents are the family of calcium blocking agents which may be able to alter the "no-reflow" phenomenon seen in cerebral blood flow following cardiac arrest. While experiments in our laboratory [13] have shown lidoflazine does not imrpove cerebral blood flow following global cerebral ischemia, this is not the end of the story. The future in this area is in the physiologic and pharmacologic mating of information in cardiac and cerebral blood flow. It is an exciting and stimulating time in the field.

REFERENCES

1. Schiff M: Ueber direkte Reizung der Herzoberflache. Arch Ges Physiol 28:200, 1982.

2. Kouwenhoven WB, Jude JR, Knickerbocker GG: Closed-chest cardiac massage. JAMA 173:1064, 1960.

3. Criley JM, Blarfuss AH, Kissel GL: Cough-induced cardiac compression. JAMA 263:1246, 1976.

4. Rudikoff MT, Maughan WL, Effron M, Freund P, Weisfeldt ML: Mechanism of blood flow during cardiopulmonary resuscitation. Circulation 61:345, 1980.

5. Weisfledt ML, Chandra N, Tsitlik J: Increased intrathoracic pressure not direct heart compression - causes the rise in intra-thoracic vascular pressures during CPR in dogs and pigs. Crit Care Med 9:377, 1981.

6. Koehler RC, Chandra N, Guerci AD, Tsitlik J, Traystman RJ, Rogers MC, Weisfeldt ML: Augmentation of cerebral perfusion by simultaneous chest compression and lung inflation with abdominal binding following cardiac arrest in dogs. Circulation 67:266, 1983.

7. Chandra N, Weisfeldt ML, Tsitlik J, Vaghaiwalla F, Snyder LD, Hoffecker M, Rudikoff MT: Augmentation of carotid flow during CPR by ventilation at high airway pressure simultaneous with chest compression. Am J Cardiol 48:1053, 1981.

8. Chandra N, Rudikoff M, Weisfeldt ML: Simultaneous chest compression and ventilation at high airway pressure during cardiopulmonary resuscitation. Lancet 1:175, 1980.

9. Shapiro HM, Marshall LF: Intracranial pressure responses to PEEP in head-injured patients. J Trauma 18:254, 1978.

10. Luce JM, Huseby JS, Kirk W, Butler J: Mechanisms by which positive endexpiratory pressure increases cerebrospinal fluid pressure in dogs. J Appl Physiol: Respir Environ Exercise Physiol 52:231, 1982.

11. Rogers MC, Nugent SK, Stidham GL: Effects of closed-chest cardiac massage in intracranial pressure. Crit Care Med 7:454, 1979.

REFERENCES

12. Michael JR, Guerci AD, Koehler RC, Shi AY, Tsitlik J, Chandra N, Niedermeyer E, Rogers MC, Traystman RJ, Weisfeldt, ML: Mechanisms whereby epinephrine augments cerebral and myocardial perfusion during cardiopulmonary resuscitation in dogs. Circulation 69: 822, 1984.
13. Dean, JM, Hoehner, PJ, Rogers, MC, Traystman, RJ: Effect of lidoflazine on cerebral blood flow following 12 minutes of total cerebral ischemia. Stroke 15:531, 1984.

THE CARDIOVASCULAR EFFECTS OF INHALATIONAL ANESTHETICS

M.K. CAHALAN, MD

All anesthetists appreciate that inhalational anesthetics may produce profound cardiovascular effects. These "side effects" are generally dose dependent and can often be used to benefit patients.

1. MYOCARDIAL CONTRACTILITY

To isolate an anesthetic's effect on contractility from confounding effects on afterload, preload, and heart rate, investigators have used in vitro preparations to show that 1 MAC of enflurane, isoflurane, or halothane produces substantial (from 10 to 40%) decreases in the maximum velocity and force of contraction of an isolated strip of cardiac muscle.[1-3] In experiments on volunteers, Eger et al.[4] and Calverly et al.[5] found indirect evidence of myocardial depression with halothane and enflurane: decreased blood pressure and cardiac output, with modest increases in right atrial pressure. Ballistocardiographic studies conducted by these investigators showed that halothane and enflurane decreased the vigor of ejection of blood from the heart. In contrast, Stevens et al. found evidence for preservation of myocardial contractility during isoflurane anesthesia: preservation of cardiac output, right atrial pressure, and the vigor of ejection of blood from the heart.[6] However, these indirect measures of myocardial contractility are also functions of afterload, preload, and heart rate. Beaupre et al. compared the effects of the three vapors at 1 and 1.5 MAC during surgery.[7] He demonstrated that velocity of circumferential fiber shortening decreased when the anesthetic level increased while afterload (systolic wall stress) remained unchanged or also decreased. Preload and heart rate did not change, and the combination of these events proves that all three of the agents result in significant myocardial depression.

We all appreciate that the modest level of myocardial depression experienced by our healthy patients during routine anesthetics is of little clinical significance. But, what about patients with failing hearts? Kemmotsu et al. examined this question in regard to isoflurane.[2] He utilized the muscle bath to demonstrate that at comparable isoflurane exposures, muscles obtained from animals with congestive heart failure were depressed to a greater degree than those obtained from animals with normal hearts. Thus, some scientific foundation exists for the widely held tenet that patients with poor ventricular function should not receive halothane, enflurane, or isoflurane. Reiz et al. investigated this question in ten patients with documented congestive heart failure.[8] He found that 1% end-tidal halothane decreased mean arterial pressure 43%, systemic vascular resistance 31%, cardiac output 20%, left ventricular work 62%, and pulmonary artery occlusion pressure 42%. None of his patients experienced myocardial ischemia although most had coronary artery disease. Indeed, his patients tolerated this anesthetic approach so well because halothane "unloaded" the ventricle more than it depressed it. Patients with congestive heart failure often receive diuretics, and the combination of the disease process and treatment may result in high peripheral vascular resistance. When exposed to inhalational anesthetic, the peripheral vasoconstriction relaxes, left ventricular work decreases, and satisfactory hemodynamics result. Comparable studies for enflurane and isoflurane are not yet available, but because of their inherent vasodilating characteristics, I suspect they will prove equally beneficial.

However, myocardial depression is a dose related phenomenon even in healthy hearts, and the safe range of anesthetic concentrations for patients with compromised ventricular function may be narrow. Certainly patients with congestive heart failure develop higher end-tidal concentrations of the vapors at any given inspired concentration than patients without failure. Therefore, we must conclude that the inhalational vapors are myocardial depressants, but that depression is of minimal consequence in normal hearts and may be well tolerated (albeit in somewhat lower doses) in failing hearts.

2. HEART RATE

In young healthy volunteers not subjected to surgery, enflurane and isoflurane increase heart rate 20 to 40%, but halothane does not.[4-6] All three vapors produce 30 to 40% decreases in mean arterial pressure. Because a high heart rate and low blood pressure can cause myocardial ischemia, the hemodynamic alterations reported for enflurane and isoflurane may not be tolerated in all surgical patients. However, in adult surgical patients receiving enflurane or isoflurane at the University of California, San Francisco, we have noted smaller increases in heart rate. In fact, we have observed that decreases in heart rate occur when morphine is given before, or fentanyl during, anesthesia with any of the three vapors. To test these clinical observations, we performed a study in which 88 healthy adult patients scheduled for elective surgery participated.[9] When we gave no narcotics, we found data similar to that from the volunteer studies -- similar in direction, but different in magnitude. Enflurane and isoflurane caused a 5 to 10% increase in heart rate, while halothane caused no change. However, if 1 mcg/Kg (about 1.5 ml) of fentanyl was given, this increase was reversed and the heart rate fell to below the preinduction value. When 0.15 mg/Kg of morphine was given as premedication, these changes were prevented altogether. But, in our study, the patients who received narcotics generally had lower blood pressures than patients in comparable anesthetic groups who did not receive narcotics. Note, however, that the decrease in heart rate was proportionally larger than the decrease in blood pressure and one would expect the balance of myocardial oxygen supply and demand to be favorably influenced. Therefore, for patients in whom modest increases in heart rate may be deleterious, morphine premedication may be advantageous if volatile anesthetics are to be used. If increases in heart rate during surgery require treatment, a small dose of fentanyl should be viewed as a possibly effective therapy. Usually, a tachycardia occurring during anesthesia and surgery has an explanation other than the anesthetic agent.

3. BLOOD PRESSURE

All three of the inhalational vapors decrease blood pressure in a dose related fashion.[4-6] The studies in volunteers suggest that enflurane may produce greater decreases in blood pressure than isoflurane or halothane, but in these studies the individuals were not stimulated by ongoing surgery and thus the blood pressure decreases were pronounced.

Nitrous oxide has little effect on arterial blood pressure even when it is administered in concentrations sufficient to induce anesthesia (studies conducted in a hyperbaric chamber).[10] One can maintain the same depth of anesthesia by substituting 60% nitrous oxide for a half MAC of one of the vapors, and as you would expect this technique usually results in significantly higher blood pressures. When this is done with isoflurane, cardiac output is not affected, but the decrease in peripheral vascular resistance is attenuated significantly.[11] Bahlman et al. investigated the effects of adding nitrous oxide to halothane -- oxygen anesthesia. They found a significantly higher mean arterial pressure, unchanged total peripheral resistance, and a higher cardiac output.[12] Smith et al. looked at the effects of adding nitrous oxide to enflurane -- oxygen anesthesia.[13] They did not find a significant difference in mean arterial pressure, and concluded that nitrous oxide does not stimulate the cardiovascular system in the presence of enflurane as it seems to in the presence of halothane or isoflurane. We can conclude that all three of the vapors depress blood pressure to comparable degrees (albeit by different mechanisms -- see more about this below), and nitrous oxide will attenuate that pressure decrease when substituted for some of the isoflurane or halothane.

4. CARDIAC OUTPUT

In the volunteer experiments, halothane and enflurane caused a dose related fall in cardiac output, such that, at 1 1/2 MAC cardiac output was approximately 70% of its control level.[4,5] Isoflurane, in contrast, was not associated with a significant reduction in cardiac output, even at the 2 MAC level.[6] In none of these studies did the investigators find evidence of inadequate perfusion. For instance, the change in base excess was on the order of 1-3 mEq/l at the 1.5 MAC level. However, unlike halothane and enflurane, isoflurane produces a two fold increase in blood flow to muscle beds. Other organs such as the brain, heart, kidneys, and GI tract receive comparable blood flows during anesthesia with any of the three vapors. Thus, one must question the significance of a preservation of overall cardiac output with isoflurane.

Three extreme examples are worth noting. First, in 13 patients requiring cerebral aneurysm surgery, Lam et al. used isoflurane to produce profound hypotension (MAP 40 torr) without change in cardiac output or the adequacy of tissue perfusion. Second, Newberg et al. reported that an MAP of 40 in the dog could be achieved with isoflurane without depleting CNS high energy compounds, but not when enflurane, halothane, nitroprusside, or trimethaphan were the hypotensive agents.[15] Third, Wolfson et al. used an animal model to demonstrate that the therapeutic window (the ratio of the lethal concentration to the effective concentration) is twice as great for isoflurane as it is for enflurane or halothane.[16] Perhaps, these differences are due, at least in part, to preservation of cardiac output.

Volatile anesthetics alter cerebral vascular tone, and despite decreasing systemic blood pressure, they all may cause increases in intracranial pressure. However, halothane and enflurane appear to be more potent in this regard than isoflurane, which when coupled with hyperventilation reliably results in no change or a decrease in cerebral blood flow.[15]

5. MYOCARDIAL ISCHEMIA

Our anesthetic agents seem ideally suited for patients with ischemic heart disease, since they directly decrease left ventricular work as well as the body's overall need for perfusion. Obviously, diastolic aortic pressure could fall to a level inadequate to push blood past a coronary constriction, but, in general, the work of the heart falls more than the decrease in perfusion across the stenosis.

Dr. Reiz et al. recently suggested that isoflurane may be different in this regard.[17] They found evidence of myocardial ischemia in 10 of 21 patients who had coronary artery disease and were anesthetized with isoflurane. Since he had no control groups, we do not know how other anesthetics might have fared, but such a high incidence of ischemia before the start of surgery is distressing. However, certain aspects of this elegant experiment make the results impossible to apply to our clinical practice. First, he witheld all the patients' cardiac medications (including beta blockers) and gave no premedication the morning of the anesthetic. He used inspired concentrations of oxygen sufficiently low to keep the P_aO_2 at its preinduction level. That is, he held the P_aO_2 in the 80-90 torr range during the study by administering 70-80% nitrogen. Clinical studies have not confirmed these findings. When Moffitt et al. studied 12 patients with coronary artery disease who were anesthetized with isoflurane and oxygen, he found isolated incidences of myocardial lactate production; but in general, lactate extraction continued throughout the case and ST segment changes were not seen.[18]

In our studies at U.C.S.F., we have compared the incidence of myocardial ischemia in patients undergoing carotid endarterectomy anesthetized either with halothane or isoflurane. In patients undergoing myocardial revascularization, we have compared the incidence of myocardial ischemia in patients anesthetized with fentanyl (100 mcg/Kg) and those anesthetized with fentanyl and isoflurane (15 mcg/Kg and 0.25-2% end-tidal isoflorane). In neither case did we find a disproportionately high incidence of myocardial ischemia in those patients exposed to isoflurane.

6. SUMMARY

Traditionally, the cardiovascular effects of the inhalational anesthetics have been regarded as "side effects". However, their ability to control blood pressure, reduce myocardial contractility, and prevent noxious stimuli from inducing myocardial ischemia can clearly be used to benefit our patients.

REFERENCES
1. Shimosato S, Sugai N, Iwatsuki N et al.: The effect of ethrane on cardiac muscle mechanics. Anesthesiology 30:514-518, 1969
2. Kemmotsu O, Hashimoto Y, Shimosato S: Inotropic effects of isoflurane on mechanics of contraction in isolated cat papillary muscles from normal and failing hearts. Anesthesiology 39:470-477, 1973
3. Sugai N, Shimosato S, Etsten BE: Effect of halothane on force - velocity relations and dynamic stiffness of isolated heart muscle. Anesthesiology 29:267-274, 1968
4. Eger EI II, Smith NT, Stoelting RK, et al.: Cardiovascular effects of halothane in man. Anesthesiology 32:396-409, 1970
5. Calverley RK, Smith NT, Prys-Roberts C et al.: Cardiovascular effects of enflurane anesthesia during controlled ventilation in man. Anesth Analg 57:619-628, 1978b
6. Stevens WC, Cromwell TH, Halsey MJ et al.: The cardiovascular effects of a new inhalation anesthetic, forane, in human volunteers at constant arterial carbon dioxide tension. Anesthesiology 35:8-16, 1971

7. Beaupre PN, Cahalan MK, Kremer PF, Lurz FW, Hamilton WK: Isoflurane, halothane, and enflurane depress myocardial contractility in patients undergoing surgery. Anesthesiology Suppl 59:A59, 1983
8. Reiz S, Balfors E, Gustavsson B et al.: Effects of halothane on coronary haemodynamics and myocardial metabolism in patients with ischemic heart disease and heart failure. Acta Anaesth Scand 26:133-138, 1982
9. Cahalan MK, Lurz FW, Beaupre PN, Schwartz LA, Eger EI II: Narcotics alter the heart rate and blood pressure response to inhalational anesthetics. Anesthesiology Suppl 59:A26, 1983
10. Winter PM, Hornbein TF, Smith G et al.: Hyperbaric nitrous oxide anesthesia in man: Determination of anesthetic potency (MAC) and cardiorespiratory effects. Abstracts of Scientific Papers. Annual Meeting of the American Society of Anesthesiologists, 1972, PP 103-104
11. Dolan WM, Stevens WC, Eger EI II et al.: The cardiovascular and respiratory effects of isoflurane-nitrous oxide anaesthesia. Can Anaesth Soc J 21:557-568, 1974
12. Bahlman SH, Eger EI II, Smith NT, Stevens WC, Shakespeare TF, Sawyer DC, Halsey MJ, Cromwell TH: The cardiovascular effects of nitrous oxide - halothane anesthesia in man. Anesthesiology 35:274-285, 1971
13. Smith NT, Calverley RK, Prys-Roberts C, Eger EI II, Jones CW: Impact of nitrous oxide on the circulation during enflurane anesthesia in man. Anesthesiology 48:345-349, 1978
14. Lam AM, Gelb AW: Cardiovascular effects of isoflurane-induced hypotension for cerebral aneurysm surgery. Anesth Analg 62:742-748, 1983
15. Newberg LA, Milde JH, Michenfelder JD: Systemic and cerebral effects of isoflurane-induced hypotension in dogs. Anesthesiology 60:541-546, 1984
16. Wolfson B, Hetrick WD, Lake CL, Siker ES: Anesthetic indices - further data. Anesthesiology 48:187-190, 1978
17. Reiz S, Balfors E, Sorensen MB et al.: Isoflurane a powerful coronary vasodilator in patients with coronary artery disease. Anesthesiology 59:91-97, 1983
18. Moffitt EA, Barker RA, Glenn JJ et al.: Myocardial metabolism and hemodynamic responses with isoflurane anesthesia for coronary artery surgery. Anesth Analg 63:175-284, 1984

CARDIAC MONITORING TECHNIQUES OF THE FUTURE: TRANSESOPHAGEAL 2-D ECHOCARDIOGRAPHY

M.K. CAHALAN, MD

During the last decade, advancements in the field of echocardiography have been so rapid that few physicians are aware of all the potential applications of this discipline.[1] Numerous studies in both humans and animals now document that 2-D echocardiography can accurately quantitate left ventricular filling and ejection.[2-5] Perhaps more importantly, it can detect episodes of myocardial ischemia before or in the absence of detection by our other clinical monitors.[6,7] Within seconds after the onset of myocardial ischemia, the affected area of muscle ceases to contract and may actually move paradoxically (outward instead of inward during systole). Thus the sudden development of a segmental wall motion abnormality is virtually pathognomonic for myocardial ischemia.

After the introduction of transesophageal 2-D echocardiography by researchers in West Germany,[8] we were given the opportunity to collaborate with them to study this technique for intraoperative cardiac monitoring. We use a commercially available phased array, 3.5 megahertz transducer system (Diasonics) consisting of 32 linearly arranged piezoelectric elements mounted on the tip of a gastroscope. The transducer is 35 mm long, 15 mm wide and 16 mm thick. An acoustical lens within the plastic mounting of the transducer focuses the ultrasound beam 2 to 15 cm in front of the array. With appropriate phasing of the single elements by a Diasonics 3400R or CV60 ultrasonograph, a 90 degree sector for real time imaging is obtained. Although no morbidity or mortality has ever been shown to result from echocardiographic studies, this system is by no means free. Approximately $60,000 would be required to purchase it, but the probe is reusable for an indefinite number of cases. We substitute this instrument for the esophageal stethoscope and thus the patient does not undergo an additional esophageal instrumentation.

After the transducer has been inserted through the mouth and advanced about 35 to 40 cm, both ventricles, the mitral and aortic valves, and the left atrium can be viewed. The juxtaposition of the left ventricular outflow track, aortic valve, and mitral valve can also be observed. Advancing the transducer another 2 to 5 cm (and angling it forward) allows cross sectional images of the left ventricle, including a short axis view at the level of the papillary muscles. If the heart is not enlarged, cross-sectional views of both ventricles frequently can be obtained.

With approval from our Commttee on Human Experimentation and informed consent from each patient, we have studied over 350 patients to determine the efficacy and usefulness of this monitoring technique. We obtained high resolution echocardiograms in 98% of our patients and no complications have resulted.[9] Inserting and positioning the ultrasound transducer usually requires less than 60 seconds. We monitor the short axis view of the left ventricle at the level of the papillary muscles and have done so for up to 12 hours. We have observed intraoperative changes in left ventricular filling, wall motion, and intravascular air. Quantitative estimates of left ventricular filling and ejection could be produced by the same observer to within 10% and by different observers to within 15%. This information was often unavailable from standard intraoperative monitors and occasionally was decisive for the care of the patient.

Three of our recently completed studies indicate that 2-D transesophageal echocardiography may provide significant advantages over our customary intraoperative monitors. In the first, we studied 32 ASA III or IV patients scheduled for major vascular or cardiac surgery.[10] At predetermined times during the surgery, we made simultaneous recordings of the pulmonary capillary wedge pressure and the 2-D echocardiogram. After demonstrating that changes in left ventricular end diastolic volume could be consistently detected by the echocardiograms, we compared these determinations with the changes in pulmonary capillary wedge pressure. In 77 % of the patients, virtually no correlation existed between changes in pulmonary capillary wedge pressure and changes in left ventricular end diastolic filling. Fifty-four percent of the patients had either large increases in filling with no change in pulmonary capillary wedge pressure or significant increases in the wedge pressure with no changes in left ventricular filling. We concluded that 2-D transesophageal echocardiography can provide consistent estimates of changes in left ventricular end diastolic filling and that the use of pulmonary capillary wedge pressure as a guide to intraoperative changes in left ventricular volumes may be misleading.

In the second study we examined a similar group of 43 high risk patients.[11] Again, at predetermined intervals during surgery, we recorded the echocardiograms on videotape. These images were evaluated by an echocardiographer who had no knowledge of the clinical outcomes. For each patient, he determined one of three results: no new regional contraction abnormalities developed, transient abnormalities developed but resolved prior to the last interval (skin closure), or new abnormalities developed and persisted through the last interval. All patients in this study had serial postoperative EKG and cardiac isoenzyme studies.

Eight patients experienced transient left ventricular regional contraction abnormalities and none of these patients went on to have a myocardial infarction. Seven patients developed persistent left ventricular regional contraction abnormalities and five of these patients developed a myocardial infarction. The distribution of the myocardial infarction could be predicted in every case by the distribution of the persistent contraction abnormality detected by the intraoperative echocardiograms. No patient who failed to develop a regional contraction abnormality later developed evidence of an intraoperative or postoperative myocardial infarction. We concluded from this study that 2-D transesophageal echocardiography may help predict which patients will suffer postoperative myocardial infarctions.

In a subsequent study, we compared the efficacy of a multilead ECG system and the 2-D transesophageal echocardiographic system for the detection of intraoperative myocardial ischemia.[12] In 50 patients undergoing either vascular or cardiac surgery, five patients developed ST segment changes of one mm or greater during induction of anesthesia (all of these changes reverted to baseline within minutes following endotracheal intubation). No transesophageal echocardiograms were available during this time, because the probe is not placed until after endotracheal intubation. During surgery six different patients developed ST segment changes. Using the first echocardiogram as the control (obtained after intubation) we documented the development of new segmental wall motion abnormalities in 24 patients. All six patients who had intraoperative ST segment changes also had segmental wall motion abnormalities. In three of these patients the change in segmental wall motion preceded the change on the electrocardiogram. Four patients who had segmental wall motion abnormalities had conduction abnormalities which precluded ECG interpretation. One patient with a segmental wall motion abnormality during left bundle branch block continued to have segmental wall motion abnormalities after conduction normalized, without ST segment abnormality. In 339 of 350 intervals we attempted to record, adequate echocardiograms were actually obtained. In only one patient were we unable to obtain the appropriate left ventricular cross-sectional view at any time during the case. Four patients had perioperative myocardial infarctions: three had persistent segmental wall motion abnormalities, while only one had a persistent ST segment change. An additional eight patients with persistent segmental wall motion abnormalities and two with persistent changes on the ECG did not suffer myocardial infarctions. One patient who suffered a myocardial infarction without having experienced a persistent intraoperative segmental wall motion abnormality or ECG change (he did have a transient segmental wall motion abnormality but no ECG changes) had his infarction not intraoperatively but three days postoperatively. We concluded from this study that the 2-D echo provides a more sensitive method for detecting intraoperative myocardial ischemia and impending infarction than the ECG.

Echocardiography can detect small quantities of intravascular air. Cardiac surgery and certain neurosurgical procedures permit entry of air into the circulation. Moreover, 2-D transesophageal echocardiography provides a nearly ideal vantage from which to view the intra-atrial septum, and contrast studies during 2-D transesophageal echocardiography can reliably diagnose atrial septal defects.[13] Thus 2-D transesophageal echocardiography is not only a sensitive detector of intravascular air, but is also the first intraoperative monitor that can identify patients at risk for experiencing paradoxical emboli.

Cucchiara et al. studied 12 patients who were to undergo suboccipital craniotomy in a sitting position.[14] He monitored these patients with both the

2-D transesophageal echocardiogram and a precordial Doppler unit. All eight cases of Doppler detected air were visualized by the transesophageal echocardiograms. In two of the cases, air was noted first on the echocardiogram. In two more cases, a questionable Doppler change was noted and the air was verified by the echocardiograms. In one severe episode of air embolization, air could be seen crossing from the right to left atrium and passing to the left ventricle and aorta. Of course, the precordial Doppler did not detect this event. These investigators concluded that the two dimensional echocardiogram was at least as sensitive as the precordial Doppler in detecting air embolization and probably more so.

Severe intraoperative hemodynamic instability may result from inadequate left ventricular filling volumes or impaired myocardial contraction. The treatments of these causes of instability may have effects that are diametrically opposed. Although use of a pulmonary artery catheter would probably give the correct diagnosis in most cases, sufficient qualitative information is immediately obvious from 2-D transesophageal echocardiography, and the introduction of the 2-D transesophageal transducer into the esophagus is inherently less hazardous than pulmonary artery catheterization.

Clearly, two-dimensional transesophageal echocardiography has promise as a less invasive and more informative method of intraoperative cardiac monitoring. However, many problems must be resolved before this technique could be instituted as a clinical tool. Mass production would almost certainly reduce its expense to less than that of pulmonary artery catheterization. The addition of quantitative transesophageal Doppler techniques will allow us to determine cardiac output and transvalvular pressure gradients. But, these efforts will not be enough. Before we launch another multimillion dollar perioperative monitoring endeavor we must demonstrate that this technique truly can be made to benefit our patients.

Monitoring techniques will change. Each new approach will offer inherent advantages and disadvantages. Our patients grow less and less tolerant of "unfortunate" outcomes and expect us to prevent them. Because iatrogenic injury is so repugnant to us all, the future belongs to the least invasive techniques which will dependably and affordably provide us with the necessary information. If we as a specialty make the correct decisions, then forces external to medicine may not be compelled to interfere.

REFERENCES

1. Popp RL, Rubenson DS, Tucker CR, French JW: Echocardiography: M-mode and two-dimensional methods. Ann Int Med 93:844-856, 1980
2. Starling MR, Crawford MH, Sorensen SG et al.: Comparative accuracy of apical biplane cross-sectional echocardiography in gated equilibrium radionucleide angiography for estimating left ventricular size and performance. Circulation 63:1075-1084, 1981
3. Tortoledo FA, Quinones MA, Fernandez GC et al.: Quantification of left ventricular volumes by two-dimensional echocardiography: a simplified and accurate approach. Circulation 67:579-584, 1983
4. Folland ED, Parisi AF, Moynihan PF et al.: Assessment of left ventricular ejection fraction and volumes by real time, two-dimensional echocardiography. A comparison of cineangeographic and radionucleide techniques. Circulation 60:760-766, 1979
5. Schiller NB, Acquatella H, Ports TA et al.: Left ventricular volume from paired biplane two-dimensional echocardiography. Circulation 60:547-555, 1979
6. Battler A, Froelicker VF, Gallagher KP et al.: Dissociation between regional myocardial dysfunction and ECG changes during ischemia in the conscious dog. Circulation 62:735-744, 1981
7. Horowitz RS, Morganroth J, Parroto C et al.: Immediate diagnosis of acute myocardial infarction by two-dimensional echocardiography. Circulation 65:323-329, 1982
8. Schluter M, Langenstein BA, Polster J et al.: Transesophageal cross-sectional echocardiography with a phased array transducer system. Technique and additional clinical results. Br Heart J 48:67-72, 1982
9. Cahalan MK, Kremer PF, Beaupre PN et al.: Consistency and reproducibility of transesophageal two-dimensional echocardiography. Anesth Analg 63:194, 1984
10. Beaupre PN, Cahalan MK, Kremer PF et al.: Does pulmonary artery occlusion pressure adequately reflect left ventricular filling during anesthesia in surgery? Anesthesiology 59:A3, 1983
11. Cahalan MK, Kremer PF, Beaupre PN et al.: Intraoperative myocardial ischemia detected by transesophageal two-dimensional echocardiography. Anesthesiology 59:A164, 1983
12. Smith JS, Benefiel DJ, Lurz FW et al.: Detection of intraoperative myocardial ischemia: ECG versus 2-d transesophageal echocardiography. Anesthesiology (abstract in press)
13. Thier W, Schluter M, Kremer P et al.: Transesophageal two-dimensional echocardiography: better demonstration of intraatrial structures. Deutsche Medizinische Wochenschrift 108:1903-1907, 1983
14. Cucchiara RF, Nugent M, Seward J, and Messick JM: Detection of air embolism in upright neurosurgical patients by 2-D transesophageal echocardiography. Anesthesiology 59:83-88, 1983

NON-INVASIVE MONITORING: IN VIVO BIOCHEMISTRY

MARK C. ROGERS, M.D.

With development of new technology, monitoring techiques have undergone substantial changes over the last two decades. The ability to use computers and the ability to miniaturize equipment have meant that we have produced major developments since our original monitoring techniques during anesthesia. This has occurred both in the sophistication of the observations -- now a long way beyond simple pulse, respiration, and blood pressure -- as well as the frequency of monitoring -- now second-by-second instead of in five minute intervals. As we move further along, we can anticipate that the variables which we monitor will likewise become even more sophisticated and more frequent.

As an example, we have become more concerned regarding the adequacy of oxygenation. Historically, we began with simple hemodynamic measurements such as blood pressure and pulse, and have moved to filling pressures of the various cardiac chambers and to cardiac output measurements by Swan Ganz catheter. None of these relate directly to the adequacy of oxygenation and do not replace simple observation of patient color. While invasive monitoring of arterial blood gases does offer the potential for monitoring oxygenation, it is invasive and in large numbers of patients the complications do not warrant the risk. As a result, there has been a growth of interest in the ability to do noninvasive monitoring of oxygenation. Most of us are familiar with the technique by which oxygen saturation of hemoglobin is measured in the catherization laboratory and perhaps with even the newer technology of fingertip sensing of oxygen saturation. This concept may be thought of as a general area of infrared spectroscopy, a noninvasive metabolic monitoring technique likely to expand in the future. This review will concentrate on some newer thoughts in which infrared spectroscopy may be useful with an eye toward how patients will be monitored in the operating room and the intensive care units in the future.

INFRARED SPECTROSCOPY

Many technologies expose a part of the patient's body to electromagnetic radiation and monitor the outcome. The electromagnetic radiation itself may be transmitted through the body with no effect, may be reflected, or may be scattered. The result is that either the radiation is passed through the body or is absorbed with a release of heat, change of wave length, or photochemical reaction. Regardless, a classic example of the usefulness of this technique is found in the use of x-rays. With this form of radiation, the energy is so high that it penetrates body tissues and is transmitted to the film opposite. New technologies, including infrared spectroscopy, deal with low energy, low frequency radiation which are considered to be "noninvasive."

Infrared and near infrared light (700 to 1,000 nm) can be useful for monitoring tissues in organs within the body because, unlike visible light these wave lengths penetrate fairly well even through bone. Furthermore, there are important molecules with absorption bands in the spectrum. In particular, hemoglobin, both oxygenated and unoxygenated, as well as portions of the cytochromes system have absorption bands in the spectrum. For instance, the oxidized form of cytochrome a,a_3 has one absorption band at 820 to 840 nm. This cytochrome is the final reaction in the respiratory chain and accounts for 90% of all cellular oxygen utilization. Measurement of this compound is useful to determine physiologic function within cells and the ability of the cells appropriately utilize oxygen. As a result, infrared monitoring has the potential for obtaining an integrated picture of oxygen supply and intracellular oxygen utilization. It even can be used to observe changes in organ blood volume by adding the amount of oxygenated and unoxygenated hemoglobin in the field.

BASIC THEORY OF INFRARED TRANSMISSION THROUGH BIOLOGIC TISSUE

There have been numerous uses of the transmission, reflection and scattering characteristics of hemolized and whole blood for the determination of blood oxygen content. Van Assendelft[1] et al, have used in vitro methods for the determination of blood oxygenation and Polanyi and Hehir[2]

used an _in vivo_ method with an indwelling fiberoptic catheter. Millikan[3] describes an ear oximeter which is, in theory, very close to the whole head oximetry method of Jobsis[4] whose method we will discuss in detail.

The ability of blood and body tissue to allow transmission of light varies from extremely low value at the blue end of the spectrum to a low, but definite, value at the red end of the spectrum. This can easily be demonstrated by shining a flashlight through your hand; the transmitted light is very red in color. This is mainly due to the increase in blood transmission in the red and near infrared. When light is transmitted through the hand, for example, there is a large scattered component; the light seen coming through is very diffuse. For measurement of blood oxygenation content by transmission, the visible spectrum is often employed[3] taking advantage of the several isobestic points between 500 and 600 nm where the transmission is independent of blood oxygen content, i.e., both oxygenated and deoxygenated blood have the same transmission.

At 805 nm there is a second isobestic point in transmission[2] and, in addition, the same isobestic wave length is present for light reflected from oxygenated and deoxygenated blood[6]. This is not true for the visible spectrum. The extinction coefficient of whole blood also decreases by almost two orders of magnitude in the near infrared from what it is in the visible[5].

When light at 805 nm is transmitted through the head, the intensity recorded is independent of blood oxygenation; it depends only on the blood and tissue transmission. If the tissue transmission is constant, then changes in signal levels represent changes in blood volume. Since the transmission of water in this region is very high[7], changes in total water volume in the head will not significantly affect the signal levels.

Since the reflectance of blood at 760 nm increases with increased oxygenation[6] and the transmission decreases[5], a change in transmitted signal at this wave length can be used as an indicator of blood oxygen content in the head. The transmitted signal level at 805 nm is a measure of total blood volume and the ratio of the signal level at 760 to that at 805 nm is a measure of blood oxygenation[8].

CLINICAL UTILITY OF THE CONCEPT

In 1977, Jobsis[4] reported that he had done some preliminary studies indicating that it was possible to measure noninvasively cerebral blood volume and what he termed "oxygen sufficiency" using the principles outlined above. In one patient with elective hyperventilation and in an unknown number of cats subjected to asphyxia, he reported changes in cerebral blood volume as measured by infrared technique which appeared to correlate with what would be expected in response to hyperventilation and asphyxia. With these early studies the data were not confirmed by independent measurements using alternative techiques, and the device described required special laboratory conditions to operate and could not really have been used in an intensive care setting. Nevertheless, it does offer a potential noninvasive method for measuring cerebral blood oxygen saturation and cerebral blood volume which is of significant potential clinical importance.

Cerebral blood volume is an important concept which is not often discussed because it currently cannot be measured directly. Nevertheless, cerebral vascular congestion can cause brain swelling and increases in intracranial pressure[12]. Furthermore, in settings most likely to result in brain edema, such as trauma or anoxic encephalopathy, there is an associated loss of cerebral autoregulation which may present a simultaneous increase in cerebral blood volume[12]. In this setting, it has been clearly shown that even minor changes in cerebral blood volume may have profound effects on intracranial pressure, cerebral perfusion pressure and cerebral blood flow[9,10,11].

Thus, it is apparent that the treatment of patients with neurologic insults includes management not only of brain edema but also with changes in cerebral blood volume produced by loss of autoregulation. Even when autoregulation is lost, however, a decrease in arterial $PaCO_2$ has been shown to lower cerebral blood volume[12,13,14,15]. As a result, the use of elective hyperventilation to lower $PaCO_2$ and lower cerebral blood volume is now standard therapy for head trauma[16], Reye's syndrome, drowning[17], anoxic encephalopathy[18], refractory meningitis and a large number of other conditions. Unfortunately, there exists no technique for following the changes in cerebral blood volume produced by hyperventilation. In its place, it has been necessary to develop invasive measurements of intracranial pressure which include the placement of catheters into the ventricle[19]. All of these techniques are associated with morbidity and mortality. The ability clinically to measure changes in blood volume in a repetitive fashion would give an objective and noninvasive measurement against which to test treatments such as hyperventilation.

Should infrared measurements of total cerebral blood volume prove clinically useful, subsequent studies can be expected to be directed at developing a clinically useful index of the state of oxygenation of hemoglobin using the differing transmission characteristics of oxygenated and deoxygenated hemoglobin at different wave lengths. Based on the data of Jobsis[4], it is possible this could be carried even further, since within the infrared spectrum to be tested cytochrome a,a_3 (cytochrome oxidase) has a weak absorption band. This cytochrome, the terminal member of the respiratory chain, reacts directly with molecular oxygen and is responsible for more than 90 percent of a cellular free energy derived from the redox reactions of the cytochrome chain. It is the ability to use infrared transmission to evaluate the amount of oxygen bound to cytochrome a,a_3 which Jobsis[4] refers to as "oxygen sufficiency." If it is indeed found to be a valid and reproducible measurement, it would also be an extremely useful way to monitor patients. Those concepts are now under experimental observation in animal models.

Recent studies in anesthetized animals have shown that when the animal is made hypoxic by turning off the respirator for three minutes, this resulted in a fall in cerebral HbO_2 as evidenced by a rise in the difference in transmission between 760 & 815 nm; a rise in cerebral blood volume shown by a smaller rise in the $Hb - HbO_2$ trace; and a decrease in the oxidation of cytochrome a,a_3 as shown by a fall in the $840 - 815$ nm curve[19,20]. In rats, bilateral ligation of the common carotid arteries led to the expected decrease in cytochrome a,a_3 oxidation, accompanied by a blood volume decrease, and a greater decrease in hemoglobin saturation. These changes were reversed by releasing the clamps within 20 minutes. Cytochrome a,a_3 then overshot into a hyperoxidation state. Other studies have shown the protective effect of hypothermia during hypoxic hypotension has been demonstrated by infrared. Rats kept at body temperatures of

22°C lesser reductions in HBO2 and oxidized cytochrome a,a_3, as well as a better survival rate, than those kept at 38°C during thirty minutes of reduction in blood pressure and inspired oxygen[21].

Application to the larger human head requires an adequate light source and better detection. Using a photon counter and human volunteers, Jobsis showed that hyperventilation produced the expected increase in transmission at 815 nm, representing a decreased absoption and a decrease in Hb – HbO_2 or a decrease in cerebral blood volume[22]. Breathing 92% O2, 8% CO2 resulted in an increased blood volume measurement and a slight increase in the measurement of cytochrome a,a_3 oxidation.

Additional developments in equipment and method are needed before the technique for application can be used in the clinical area. Photon counting is difficult in the presence of extraneous light. Furthermore, while the preliminary work was conducted by transillumination, with the source and the detector along the same axis. Reflectance techniques, with the source and the detector closer to each other and not in the same axis, may help in improving signal intensity. This cannot be done until the effects of varying probe placement have been worked out. There remain some doubts as to which are the best and most reproducible wave lengths to use, especially the isobestic point for Hb – HBO_2 which affects the measurement of cerebral blood volume and the correction factor for the other two measurements. It also has not been established whether the changes in OD are linearly related to changes in amounts of these substances. Nevertheless, infrared methodology appears to be a significant breakthrough in noninvasive _in vivo_ biochemical monitoring.

REFERENCES

1. Van Assendelft: Spectrophotometry of Hemoglobin Derivatives, Thomas, Springfield, IL, 1970.

2. Polanyi, M.L. and Hehir, R.: In vivo oximeter with fast dynamic response. Rev. Sci. Inst. 33:1050-1054, 1962.

3. Millikan, G.A.: The oximeter; an instrument for measuring continuously the oxygen saturation of arterial blood in man. Rev. Sci. Inst. 13:434-444, 1942.

4. Jobsis, S: Noninvasive monitoring of cerebral and myocardial oxygen sufficiency and circulatory parameters. Science 198: 1264-1266, 1977.

5. Strong, J.: Procedures in Experimental Physics, Prentice-Hall, New York, 1952.

6. Falholt, W. Spectrophotometry on whole blood, Scan. J. Clin. Invest. 7:49-54, 1955.

7. Sklar, F.H., Burke, E.F. and Langfitt, T.W.: Cerebral blood volume: valves obtained with ^{15}Cr-labeled red blood cells and RISA. J. Appl. Physiol. 24:79-82, 1968.

8. Dubowski, K.M.: Measurements of Hemoglobin Derivatives, Lippincott, Philadelphia, PA, 1964.

9. Ahapiro, H.M.: Intracranial hypertension. Anesthesiology 43:445-471, 1975.

10. Langfitt, T.W., Weinstein, J.D. and Kassell, N.F.: Cerebral vasomotor paralysis produced by intracranial hypertension. Neurology 15:622-641, 1965.

11. Langfitt, T.W.: Increased intracranial pressure. Clin. Neurosurg. 16:436-471, 1979.

12. Smith, A.L., Neufield, G.R., Ominsky, A.J., et al: Effect of arterial CO_2 tension on cerebral blood flow, mean transit time, and vascular volume. J. Appl. Physiol. 31:701-707, 1971.

13. Grubb, R.L., Raichle, M.E., Eichling, J.O., et al: The effects of changes in $PaCO_2$ on cerebral blood volume, blood flow, and vascular mean transit time. Stroke 5:630-639, 1974.

REFERENCES

14. Phelps, M.E., Grubb, R.L. and Ter-Pogossian, M.M.: In vivo regional cerebral blood volume by x-ray fluorescence. J. Appl. Physiol. 35:741-747, 1973.

15. Grubb, R.L., Phelps, M.E. and Ter-Pogossian, M.M.: Regional cerebral blood volume in humans. Arch. Neurol. 28:38-44, 1973.

16. Rogers, M.C.: Management of intracranial pressure. Johns Hopkins Med. J. 142:99-104, 1978.

17. Nugent, S.L. and Rogers, M.C.: Resuscitation and intensive care monitoring following immersion hypothermia. J. Trauma 20: 814, 1980.

18. Nugent. S.K., Bausher, J.A., Moxon, E.R. and Rogers, M.C.: Management of raised intracranial pressure in meningitidis meningoecephalitis. Amer. J. Dis. Child. 133:260-264, 1979.

19. Caniano, D.A., Nugent, S.K., Rogers, M.C., et al: Intracranial pressure monitoring in the management of the pediatric trauma patient. J. Ped. Surg. 15:537, 1980.

20. Kariman, K., Jobsis, F.F., Saltzman, H.A.: Cytochrome a,a$_3$ Reoxidation - Early indicator of metabolic recovery from hemorrhagic shock in rats. J. Clin. Invest. 72:180, 1983.

21. Jobsis, F.F.: Noninvasive infrared monitoring of cerebral oxygen sufficiency and hemodynamic parameters. p. 223. In Popp, A.J., Ed.: Neural Trauma. Raven Press, New York, 1979.

22. Kubicek, W.G., Karnegis, J.N., Patterson, R.P. et al.: Development and evolution of an impedance cardiac output system. Aerospace Med. 37: 1208, 1966.

ANALGESIA FOR LABOR: PAST, PRESENT AND FUTURE

GERARD W. OSTHEIMER, M.D.

History (The Past) Dr. Crawford Long had participated in "ether frolics" when he was a medical student at the University of Pennsylvania. He entered practice in Jefferson, Georgia and was consulted by one of his friends, James Venable, who had two small tumors on his neck. Long persuaded Venable to have one of the tumors removed while under the influence of ether on March 30, 1842. This was the first utilization of ether for a surgical procedure. Dr. Long subsequently published an account of his use of ether in the December 1849 issue of the Southern Medical and Surgical Journal. However, Morton's work had been previously reported by Bigelow and Warren in the Boston Medical and Surgical Journal in 1846. Morton had administered ether to Gilbert Abbott so that John Collins Warren could perform a procedure on his neck on October 6, 1846. Warren and his associate, Bigelow, were largely responsible for promoting the utilization of ether to produce anesthesia for surgery.

On January 19, 1847, Sir James Y. Simpson supervised the administration of ether to produce analgesia during labor and delivery. Dr. Long may have preceeded Dr. Simpson in this use. Dr. Nathan Colley Keep administered ether for obstetric analgesia on April 7, 1847 under the guidance of Dr. Walter Channing who was the founder of the Boston Lying-In Hospital and Professor of Mid-Wifery and Medical Jurisprudence at Harvard Medical School.

Dr. Channing cut the umbilical cord and could not smell ether on the severed end, therefore, he felt ether did not go across the placenta to the fetus. However, John Snow, the first physician anesthesiologist, detected ether on the exhaled breath of the newborn, thereby demonstrating placental transfer of an inhalation agent for the first time.

Dr. Simpson's work with inhalation analgesia was greeted with some hostility in Scotland. Clergy and physicians held that pain in labor was will of God and might be beneficial to the parturient.

This feeling originates from the Bible (Genesis 3:16) "In sorrow thou shalt bring forth children". Simpson's contention was that the true meaning of this phrase had been lost in translation and that it was perfectly reasonable to administer pain relief to the parturient during labor and delivery. After Queen Victoria was given chloroform at the birth of her eighth child, Prince Leopold , by John Snow who administered it intermittently with uterine contractions, utilization of inhalation analgesia became firmly established.

In 1848, Walter Channing published a "Treatise on Etherization in Childbirth" and described his first 581 cases. I will quote from his preface: "My great, I had almost said my sole, object in this circular, - in short, in my whole efforts - was to ascertain here at home, in the birthplace of etherization, what had been the precise results of many experiments, made by many physicians, of the employment of the remedy of pain. My object was to learn if this use of it has been safe, safe both to mother and to child; and thus, as far as such results might reach, to contribute something towards settling the most important point concerning its further use, namely, that of its safety."

These principles set forth by Channing for the safety of mother and child is exactly what we are attempting to do 140 years later.

In order to understand the utilization of pain relief during labor and delivery it is essential to review the physiologic changes in the parturient and the present controversies.

Physiologic Considerations in the Parturient
A. Alterations in the Gastrointestinal System (The Present)

During pregnancy, progesterone decreases gastrointestinal motility and relaxes the gastroesophageal sphincter mechanism. The gravid uterus mechanically obstructs the duodenum and increases intragastric pressure. There may be an increase in gastric acidity secondary to stimulation of the parietal cells. During labor there is a diminution in gastric emptying with the accumulation of gastric juice and gas. These conditions greatly increase the risk of regurgitation. In the most recent report on Confidential Enquiries into Maternal Deaths in England and Wales 1976-78 (Tompkins et al, 1982)', 40 deaths were related to anesthesia. 14 deaths were related to the aspiration of gastric contents; over 50% of these women had received Mist. Mag. Trisil (B.P.) Therefore, particulate antacids do NOT provide the protection that has been ascribed to their use. Of special interest is the fact that difficulty with endotracheal intubation was responsible for 16 deaths overall and for 5 deaths in the group that aspirated. Ineffective cricoid pressure was noted in 5 parturients who died of aspiration.

Finally, "of the 40 deaths associated with anaesthesia all but two were judged to have had avoidable factors. Most of these were attributed to combinations of lack of knowledge, inexperience, low general standards of care in labour and poor administrative practices. There is a need to review the anaesthetic services in maternity units with the aim of providing better trained anaesthetists and of ensuring that the administrative arrangements are inherently safe for atients." The lesions of aspiration pneumonitis are caused by food particles and by liquid vomitus having a pH<2.5. No time interval between the last meal and either onset of labor or delivery can guarantee an empty stomach. Although a volume of 30 ml or greater places the parturient "at risk" (Roberts and Shirley, 1974)[2], the exact volume for each change in pH has not been defined.

CONTROVERSY: The particulate material in some antacid emulsions may be hazardous if aspirated. (Gibbs et al, 1979)[3]
Present investigations are focusing on the use of clear antacids (0.3 M sodium citrate and Bicitra[R]); parenteral medications that will alter gastric acidity and decrease gastric secretion (glycopyrrolate and cimetidine) or increase gastric emptying (metoclopramide). Regardless of the pharmacologic approach, there will be retained gastric contents during labor and delivery, therefore ALL parturients MUST be considered as having a "full stomach".

Steps to decrease the hazards of aspiration pneumonitis:
1. Nothing by mouth during labor
2. Clear antacid (0.3M sodium citrate or Bicitra[R]) - 30ml by mouth before the induction of anesthesia during labor or for delivery. If a cesarean delivery is planned for a parturient who has previously received the clear antacid, repeat the dose within the hour before surgery. 30ml is effective in raising the pH of liquid gastric contents above 3.0 within 6 minutes (personal experience) and up to 195 minutes (Gibbs et al, 1982)[4]

3. Regional anesthesia

4. Rapid and skillful induction of general anesthesia utilizing cricoid pressure (Sellick's maneuver) and endotracheal intubation.

5. Glycopyrrolate - ↓ salivary and ↓ gastric secretions

6. Metoclopramide - ↑ gastric emptying

7. Cimetidine - ↓ gastric secretions and acidity
For elective cesarean delivery, consider cimetidine - 300mg p.o. h.s.; Bicitra - 30 ml p.o. and cimetidine 300mg I.M. one hour before cesarean delivery. (Hodgkinson et al, 1982, Ostheimer et al, 1982)[5,6]

B. Alterations in the Cardiovascular System

Hematologic changes at term:

1. ↑ Plasma Volume (40-50%)

2. ↑ Erythrocyte Volume (20%)

3. ↑ Blood Volume (25-40%)

4. Hemoglobin (11-12 mg/dl)

5. Hematocrit (≈35%)

6. White blood cells (8-10,000/cumm)

7. ↑ Platelet count (≈300,000/cumm)

8. ↑ Fibrinogen (≈400-450 mg/dl)

9. ↑ Clotting factors; ↓ Fibrinolysis

10. ↓ Serum cholinesterase activity (60%)

Systematic changes:

Cardiac output increases progressively during pregnancy, reaching a level of 30-50 percent above the nonpregnant state in late pregnancy and slightly decreasing at term. The increase in cardiac output is the product of the increase in heart rate (12-15 beats per minute in the last trimester) and the increase in stroke volume which increases gradually until the last trimester. The increase in stroke volume is greater in the lateral than in the supine position as term approaches because of the decrease in venous return secondary to aortocaval compression in the supine position. Arterial blood pressure decreases somewhat because of a decrease in peripheral resistance. Venous pressure remains normal except below the venous obstruction produced by the gravid uterus where the pressure is increased. Cardiac output increases during labor and each

contraction further augments the circulating blood volume. The
hemodynamic changes that occur during aortocaval compression (supine
hypotension) are: ↓ venous return, ↓ stroke volume, ↓ cardiac output, ↑
and then ↓ in heart rate and ↓ arterial pressure.

Steps to decrease the hypotension that results from aortocaval
compression:

1. Acute hydration of the patient for vaginal delivery: 1000ml of
   crystalloid before the initiation of epidural or subarachnoid
   block. for cesarean delivery, use at least 1500ml.
2. The use of a wedge usually under the right hip to displace the
   uterus to the left (but occasionally the reverse must be used) to
   avoid the occlusive pressure of the uterus on the aorta and
   inferior vena cava.
3. Before the induction of anesthesia, blood pressure should be
   taken in the supine and lateral positions.
4. Marked supine hypotension may be a contraindication to the use of
   a major regional technique.
5. Ephedrine: In a study of pregnant ewes, ephedrine has been
   demonstrated to be the "best" vasopressor for use in that
   maternal blood pressure is increased with little change in
   uterine blood flow. (Ralston et al, 1974)[7]

CONTROVERSY: The Utilization and Efficacy of Ephedrine

The aggressive use of ephedrine to manage the maternal hypotension
that develops after the initiation of spinal or epidural anesthesia
maintains maternal and fetal/neonatal acid base homeostasis while
significantly decreasing the incidence of nausea and vomiting in the
parturient. (Datta et al, 1982, Kang et al, 1982)[8,9]

CONTROVERSY: Use of dextrose-containing solutions for acute
intra-vascular volume expansion.

Mothers who receive a large amount of dextrose during labor and
delivery (usually from acute hydration at the time of induction of
anesthesia) become hyperglycemic. As a result, the fetus becomes
hyperglycemic, hyperinsulinemic and acidotic. After delivery, the neonate
becomes hypoglycemic because of its hyperinsulinemic state. Kenepp et al
(1982)[10] have suggested that maternal dextrose infusion at elective
cesarean delivery (and, I believe, during labor) be restricted to 6g/hr.

C. Alterations in the Respiratory System:

During pregnancy there is capillary engorgement throughout the respiratory tract. Changes in the shape of the chest and the elevated positions of the diaphragm are caused by the growing uterus.
The following changes in pulmonary volumes and capacities occur:

	Non-pregnant	Change	Pregnant
TLC	4200 ml	↓	4000 ml
TV	450 ml	↑ ↑	600 ml
IC	2500 ml	↑	2650 ml
ERV	700 ml	↓ ↓	550 ml
RV	1000 ml	↓ ↓	800 ml
IRV	2050 ml	-----	2050 ml
FRC	1700 ml	↓ ↓	1350 ml
VC	3200 ml	-----	3200 ml
Diaphragm		↑ ↑	

The following respiratory changes occur at term: Respiratory rate ↑ (10%), Tidal volume ↑ (40%), Minute ventilation ↑ (50%) and Alveolar ventilation ↑ (60%).

Ventilation during labor and delivery is further increased involuntarily by pain, anxiety, and apprehension or voluntarily by the parturients trained in natural childbirth techniques. Changes in pulmonary volumes and ventilatory patterns increase gas exchange between the alveolus and maternal blood. The problems of hyperventilation, hypoventilation, and respiratory obstruction will produce hypocarbia, hypoxia, hypercarbia and respiratory acidosis faster in the gravida than in the nonpregnant female. The various analgesics and sedatives given during labor can further alter the ventilatory capability of the parturient. Induction of general anesthesia is more rapid in the parturient because of the increase in alveolar ventilation, decrease in functional residual capacity, and decrease in MAC.

Fetal Exposure to Maternally Administered Drugs

The factors that determine the exposure of the fetus to medication administered to the parturient:

A. Maternal factors
1. Absorption from different sites
2. Circulatory changes at term includes an increase of cardiac output during labor and with each contraction.
3. Plasma protein binding of drugs (Mother > Fetus)
4. Metabolism - Liver
5. Excretion - Kidney

B. Placental factors
1. Regional (uterine) blood flow - 20% of cardiac output at term
2. Transfer - in accordance with Fick's Law of Diffusion taking into account the physiochemical characteristics of the drug. Most important are: Molecular Weight (<600 daltons), Degree of Ionization and Lipid Solubility
Most drugs used in obstetric pain relief have molecular weights < 600, are unionized and are highly lipid soluble in order to pass the lipoprotein membrane.
3. Placental metabolism (?)
C. Fetal/Neonatal factors
1. Circulation (Fetal → Transitional → Neonatal)
2. Plasma protein binding (Mother > Fetus)
3. Metabolism - Liver
4. Excretion - Kidney
5. Amniotic fluid - ? role

Types of Pain Relief

A. Prepared Childbirth (and its variations)

CONTROVERSY: Hyperventilation, Stress and "Pushing"
1. Hyperventilation (maternal) will decrease maternal pCO_2 and fetal pO_2 (Motoyama et al, 1966)[11]
2. Maternal stress during labor will increase circulating catecholamines and decrease uterine blood flow. (Shnider et al, 1979)[12]
3. "Bearing down" in the second stage of labor will decrease uteroplacental blood flow. (Bassell et al, 1980)[13]

B. Parenteral Medications[14]
1. BARBITURATES

Secobarbital, pentobarbital, and amobarbital have continued to lose popularity since it has become increasingly apparent that they have prolonged depressant effects on the neonate as demonstrated by the initial Brazelton study on the effects of medication during labor and delivery. These sedative hypnotics possess no analgesic properties and, in agitated patients with pain, may produce an antianalgesic effect which further increases excitation, disorientation, and management problems.

2. TRANQUILIZERS

Promethazine, hydroxyzine, propiomazine, and promazine are commonly used to relieve anxiety during labor.

Chlorpromazine and prochlorperazine are less frequently used due to their propensity for causing hypotension secondary to their α-adrenergic effects. Hydroxyzine is rarely used in the author's institution since it cannot be administered intravenously in the United States. Although little work has been done on the previously mentioned tranquilizers, extensive investigations have been carried out on the major tranquilizer of our time, diazepam. A benzodiazepine derivative, this drug rapidly crosses the placenta and the fetal/maternal ratio approaches 1 in a few minutes. Several investigators have reported fetal/maternal drug concentrations in excess of 1 with diazepam. Its metabolism in the newborn is quite slow.

The drug and its active metabolite are detectable in significant concentrations in the newborn for up to 8 days. Neonates whose mothers have received large dosages of diazepam demonstrate hypotonia, lethargy, diminished sucking, hypothermia, and inability to respond to their environment as demonstrated by neurobehavioral assessments.

Recently, it has been demonstrated that lorazepam, a new benzodiazepine given for its tranquilizing and amnesic effects in parturients, produced the same effects as diazepam. Babies of mothers treated for hypertension and premature infants had a high incidence of low Apgar scores, need for ventilation, hypothermia, and poor suckling. In our institution, lorazepam does not have a place in obstetrics.

3. ATROPINE

Atropine is an anticholinergic drug used as premedication before induction of anesthesia. It blocks maternal vagal reflexes with increasing dosages and will decrease oropharyngeal and tracheal secretions. Since it readily crosses the placenta, fetal tachycardia has occurred following its maternal administration with a resultant decrease in beat-to-beat variability. Atropine, therefore, could mask the changes in fetal heart rate used to diagnose fetal distress. Recently, Abboud et al did not find any change in fetal heart rate or variability probably due to the lower dosage than that used in the previous studies. In our institution, atropine is only used in obstetric anesthesia where it is specifically indicated, for example, in cases of maternal bradycardia.

4. SCOPOLAMINE

Scopolamine is a belladonna alkaloid with less vagolytic action than atropine. It rapidly crosses the blood-brain barrier and the placenta. In the parturient, it produces amnesia and some sedation. However, it does not possess any analgesic properties. When used in the presence of pain, it often results in severe agitation, excitement, and loss of control. In the fetus it will produce loss of beat-to-beat variability and fetal tachycardia. The author believes that scopolamine has no place in labor and delivery due to the fact that maternal participation is desired in the delivery process. Even in known cases of intrauterine fetal death or congenital abnormalities, the tranquilizers produce a more satisfying course for the mother, her accompanying person, and her labor attendants.

5. NARCOTICS

Narcotics are still the primary form of pain relief used in obstetrics. The side effects of narcotic analgesia can be categorized as either maternal or fetal. Maternal effects include respiratory depression, orthostatic hypotension, nausea and vomiting, decreased gastric motility, and inhibition of labor during the latent phase. Fetal effects include loss of beat-to-beat variability, increased minute volume with respiratory acidosis, and neurobehavioral alterations.

Meperidine still is the most popular narcotic analgesic used during labor. Other narcotics that have been used are morphine, alphaprodine, pentazocine, and fentanyl.

Morphine, which can be administered in doses of 5-10 mg intramuscularly, or 2-3 mg intravenously, is not as popular as meperidine because at equianalgesic dosages, it is thought to produce more neonatal respiratory depression. This finding, however, has not been confirmed. Alphaprodine is a shorter-acting narcotic analgesic and is used in some centers.

Pentazocaine administered in doses of 20-30 mg intramuscularly or 10-20 mg intravenously has not achieved extensive popularity because of its psychomimetic effects. Fentanyl, administered in doses of 50-100 µg intramuscularly or 25-50 µg intravenously, is not widely used probably because of the rapid onset of respiratory depression and its shorter duration of action than meperidine.

Butorphanol, a narcotic agonist-antagonist, can be administered in doses of 1-2 mg intramuscularly or intravenously during labor. It has no advantages over meperidine except for possible lower respiratory depression when used in 3-4 mg doses. However, in our institution, our obstetricians have found that butorphanol, 1 mg intramuscularly and 1 mg intravenously produces the desired effect of narcosis plus some tranquilization that otherwise would be achieved by combining a narcotic and a tranquilizer. The effect of butorphanol is readily reversed by naloxone, if necessary.

Nalbuphine, another narcotic agonist-antagonist, can be given in doses of 10-15 mg intramuscularly. It also has been claimed to cause less respiratory depression than meperidine, although this probably does not occur until the administered dosage is greater than 20 mg.

Meperidine is commonly administered in doses of 50-100 mg intramuscularly or 10-50 mg intravenously. The peak analgesic effect will occur 40-45 minutes after intramuscular injection and 5-10 minutes after intravenous injection. Titration of dosage is the key to its intravenous use. The duration of action is 2-4 hours. Meperidine rapidly crosses the placenta, maternal and fetal equilibrium occurs within 6 minutes after intravenous injection. The half life of meperidine is 23 hours in the neonate and approximately 4 hours in the mother. Neonatal depression from a narcotic can be reversed by the administration of naloxone, a pure narcotic antagonist. The dosage is 0.01 mg/kg intramuscularly. Naloxone should not be administered to the mother just prior to delivery to prevent neonatal depression from maternal narcotic administration. Naloxone at this time will only reverse analgesia when it is needed most. Secondly, reversal of neonatal narcotic depression will be, at best, unpredictable. Thus, naloxone should be administered to the neonate after delivery only if clinically indicated.

C. THIOPENTAL

Thiopental is the induction agent most commonly used today. It crosses the placenta rapidly; the peak umbilical vein concentration occurs 1 minute after maternal administration. When the dosage is limited to 4 mg/kg, fetal outcome, as measured by Apgar score, is not affected. Delivery should not be delayed in an attempt to allow redistribution of drug because the fetal brain is exposed to only very small amounts. The concentration reaching the fetal brain is variable and no direct relationship can be made to neonatal neurobehavior.

D. KETAMINE

Ketamine is an intravenous agent that produces analgesia and a dissociative state regarded as sleep. Controversy surrounds the use of this drug in obstetrics. On one hand, it is an excellent induction agent for general anesthesia in cases where cardiovascular stability must be maintained, such as in abruptio placentae and placenta praevia. Its use as a powerful analgesic to produce pain relief at the time of delivery has been advocated. This technique is difficult and may result in general anesthesia together with its inherent problems of regurgitation and aspiration. Ketamine does not protect the laryngeal and pharyngeal reflexes in the obtunded or anesthetized mother. Hallucinations and delirium on emergence are common in unpremedicated patients.

Ketamine crosses the placenta rapidly and produces increasing neonatal depression in doses over 1.0 mg/kg. This depression has not been demonstrated with low dosage schedules of ketamine. However, since ketamine produces its dissociative state by excitation of the central nervous system could the newborn, in fact, be experiencing general central nervous system stimulation by this agent? In studies comparing thiopental and ketamine as induction agents for general anesthesia, infants whose mothers received ketamine scored better on the Scanlon Early Neonatal Neurobehavioral Scale than those who received thiopental. One would think that with general anesthesia, the newborn would have similar scores. The author believes that the pharmacologic effect of ketamine on the newborn's central nervous system is responsible for this apparent "better" score when contrasted with thiopental.

E. INHALATION ANESTHETICS

Inhalational anesthetics are divided into two categories: inhalation analgesics and inhalation anesthesias.

Inhalation analgesia is produced by the administration of low concentration of the inhalation anesthetics (nitrous oxide, halothane, enflurane, isoflurane, methoxyflurane) to provide partial relief of pain. The mother remains awake with intact laryngeal reflexes so that the risk of aspiration is minimized. Inhalation anesthesia results from the administration of higher concentrations of inhalation agents to produce maternal unconsciousness. With loss of consciousness, there is always the risk of maternal aspiration and cardiopulmonary depression.

1. NITROUS OXIDE

Marx and her associates have shown that induction to delivery (I-D) intervals greater than 15 minutes may result in "depression" (anesthesia?) of the newborn when 70 percent nitrous oxide/30 percent oxygen is used. When the I-D or uterine incision to delivery (UI-D) intervals are long or newborn depression is present, the neonate should breathe 100 percent oxygen immediately after delivery to decrease rapidly the concentration of nitrous oxide. Recent investigations have demonstrated that the UI-D interval is as important as the I-D interval. UI-D intervals greater than 3 minutes may lead to depression of the newborn secondary to altered uteroplacental perfusion.

2. HALOGENATED ANESTHETICS

The halogenated anesthetic agents (halothane, enflurane, isoflurane, and methoxyflurane) are frequently used as supplements to nitrous oxide. They have been shown to decrease maternal recall of intraoperative events, allow higher maternal and fetal PaO_2 by administration of higher concentrations of oxygen, and to increase uterine blood flow. Because of the dosage-related decrease in uterine contractility caused by these inhalational agents, it has been claimed that they might be associated with an increased postpartum blood loss. No increased blood loss has been demonstrated with halothane, enflurane, isoflurane, or methoxyflurane at cesarean delivery.

F. LOCAL ANESTHETICS

1. PHARMACOLOGY

Physicochemical Characteristics of the amide local anesthetics The molecular weights are < 600 and, in general, the higher the plasma protein binding of the drug, the higher is the lipid solubility. Fetal plasma protein binding of amide local anesthetics is less than the binding in maternal plasma.

2. METABOLISM AND EXCRETION

The basic difference between the ester and amide compounds are their metabolism and their allergic properties. The ester derivatives of benzoic acid are hydrolyzed in the plasma by pseudocholinesterases. The amide compounds undergo enzymatic degradation in the liver. The benzoic acid metabolites of procaine, tetracaine and 2-chloroprocaine are responsible for the allergic-type reactions seen with these agents. Reports of allergic responses to amide-type agents are very rare. There is no apparent cross sensitivity between the esters and the amides. The kidney is responsible for excretion of the local anesthetics and their metabolic products.

Regional Blocks

A. Paracervical Block
   1. Problems are related to the proximity of the injection site to the fetal head and paracervical plexus of blood vessels.
   2. Effects on the fetus:
      i. Direct - Central nervous system and myocardial depression
      ii. Indirect - (Secondary to uterine hypertonus and uterine artery vasoconstriction) - ↓ uterine artery blood flow produces fetal hypoxia and acidosis.
   3. Continuous fetal heart rate monitoring is mandatory if this block is used during labor.
   4. Technique of choice when combined with narcotic (fentanyl) and tranquilizer for pregnancy terminations or D & Cs for incomplete abortions.
B. Pudendal Block
   Uptake of drugs and effects are similar to epidural block
C. Subarachnoid Block
   1. Keys for use:
      i. Adequate acute hydration ($\simeq$ 1000 ml for vaginal delivery; > 1500 ml for cesarean delivery).
      ii. Induction - Right lateral position - especially for cesarean delivery.
      iii. #25 or #26g. needle.
      iv. Avoid aortocaval compression.
      v. Oxygen by face mask.
      vi. Treat hypotension immediately with a 200-300 ml bolus of crystalloid solution and/or ephedrine with increments of 10mg I.V. prn.
      vii. Minimize induction to delivery and uterine incision to delivery intervals during cesarean delivery.
   2. Effects on fetus/newborn related to duration of hypotension and subsequent altered uteroplacental perfusion.

D. Epidural Block
   1. Keys for use: Same as for subarachnoid block except for needle size
   2. Effects of labor:
      i. Initiation of block. The epidural block is usually initiated during the accelerating phase of the active stage of labor when the cervix is dilated approximately 5cm or more. However, there are many exceptions to this rule.
     ii. Segmental vs. "Complete" block
      Segmental block can be started earlier and will block the pain of uterine contractions and cervical dilatation. However, perineal pain relief (block of S_{2-4}) cannot be guaranteed for delivery and may require local infiltration, pudendal block or low subarachnoid block.
      "Complete" block ($T_{10}-S_4$) can provide complete pain relief but the incidence of hypotension is higher than segmental block and the second stage of labor from full dilatation until delivery is prolonged. Good nursing care is essential to help the parturient co-ordinate her "pushing" with her contractions and decrease the length of the second stage.

CONTROVERSY: What about the supposed decrease in uterine activity after the initiation of epidural analgesia? "Aortocaval compression is an essential factor contributing to or responsible for the temporary depression of uterine activity that has been observed by other authors after epidural injection of local anesthetic agents." (Schellenberg, 1977)[15]

   3. CONTROVERSY: The use of lumbar epidural block in toxemia of pregnancy.
     Lumbar epidural analgesia improves intervillous blood flow during in severe pre-eclampsia. (Jouppila et al, 1982)[16]

   4. Effects on the fetus/newborn are related to drug dosage; the interval from the last dose until delivery and altered uteroplacental perfusion secondary to maternal hypotension. Fetal acidosis has been associated with unusually high fetal/maternal concentration ratios of local anesthetics.

Neonatal Neurobehavior

CONTROVERSY: The effects of drugs given during labor and delivery on the fetus/newborn.

At present, there is reasonable documentation that the drugs used for pain relief during labor and delivery may produce transient neurobehavioral changes. Maternal hypotension has been shown to produce neurobehavioral changes and biochemical alterations in the newborn secondary to aortocaval compression by the gravid uterus alone or in conjunction with major regional anesthesia. Short periods of hypotension (<2 minutes) may unmask fetal compromise that can be demonstrated biochemically (Corke et al, 1982)[17] while longer periods of hypotension will produce altered neurobehavioral responses up to 48 hours after delivery. (Hollmen et al, 1978).[18] Ounsted et al (1980)[19] assessed 570 mothers and their children from birth to four years and found strong associations between the incidence of fetal distress during labor, birth asphyxia and delivery by emergency cesarean section with developmental scores that were below average. No associations were found with the type or amount of anesthesia in a subsequent analysis.

Epidural and Subarachnoid Narcotics (The Future)[20]

In the early 1970s, Hughes and others described endogenous 6-amino-acid peptides called enkephalins which have opiate-like characteristics. Receptors for these peptides were principally found in the periaqueductal gray and periventricular gray matter. Further work by Yaksh, Kitahata, and others elucidated spinal opiate receptors. These were found to lie in the substantia gelatinosa corresponding to Rexed laminae I, II, V. It is believed that the opiate action is at a presynaptic level, blocking release of the proposed neurotransmitter substance P, principally in the C and A δ fibers. As such, essentially only nociception is affected. Tendon and local reflexes, touch, motor function, and autonomic transmission are left intact.

The effectiveness of various narcotics when administered into the epidural space depends upon several factors including dural permeability, molecular shape, lipophilicity, and degree of ionization. Of these, lipophilicity and molecular shape vary the most. Fentanyl has an extended shape and the greatest lipid solubility, thus it has the most rapid onset of action. Morphine, being globular and of lower lipid solubility, has a delayed onset.

Administration of both intrathecal and epidural narcotics has met with varying success during labor. β-endorphin, one of the naturally occurring polypeptides, was one of the first to be administered intrathecally for analgesia during labor. Complete relief was obtained in minutes and no fetal effects were noted as measured by Apgar scores. Side effects related to the β-endorphin were minimal. This agent would seem ideal because it does not cross the blood-brain barrier. However, its extremely high cost makes routine use prohibitive at present. Side effects of epidural and subarachnoid narcotics are pruritus, urinary retention, nausea, vomiting and respiratory depression.

References:
1. Tompkins J, Turnbull A, Robson G, et al.: Report on Confidential Enquiries into Maternal Deaths in England and Wales 1976-1978. Her Majesty's Stationery Office, London.
2. Roberts RB, Shirley MA.: Reducing the risk of aspiration during cesarean section. Anesth Analg 53:859-868, 1974.
3. Gibbs CP, Schwartz DJ, Wynne JW, et al.: Antacid pulmonary aspiration in the dog. Anesthesiology 51:380-385, 1979.
4. Gibbs CP, Spohr L, Schmidt D.: The effectiveness of sodium citrate as an antacid. Anesthesiology 57:44-46, 1982.
5. Hodgkinson R, Glassenberg R, Joyce TH, et al.: Comparison of cimetidine (Tagamet) with antacid for safety and effectiveness in reducing gastric acidity before elective cesarean section. Anesthesiology 59:86-90, 1983.
6. Ostheimer GW, Morrison JA, Lavoie C, et al.: The effect of cimetidine on mother, newborn and neonatal neurobehavior. Anesthesiology 57:A405, 1982.
7. Ralston DH, Shnider SM, deLorimier AA.: Effects of equipotent ephedrine, metaraminol, mephentermine, and methoxamine on uterine blood flow in the pregnant ewe. Anesthesiology 40:354-370, 1974.
8. Datta S, Alper MH, Ostheimer GW, et al.: Method of ephedrine administration and nausea and hypotension during spinal anesthesia for cesarean section. Anesthesiology 56:48-80, 1982.
9. Kang YG, Aboulesh E, Caritis S.: Prophylactic intravenous ephedrine infusion during spinal anesthesia for cesarean section. Anesthesia and Analgesia 61:839-842, 1982.
10. Kenepp NB, Shelley WC, Gabbe SG, et al.: Fetal and neonatal hazards of maternal hydration with 5% dextrose before cesarean section. Lancet 1:1150-1152, 1982.
11. Motoyama EK, Rivard G, Acheson F, et al.: Adverse effects of maternal hyperventilation on the fetus. Lancet 1:286-288, 1966.
12. Shnider SM, Wright RG, Levinson, et al.: Uterine blood flow and plasma norepinephrine changes during maternal stress in the pregnant ewe. Anesthesiology 50:524-527, 1979.
13. Bassell GM, Humayan SG, Marx GF.: Maternal bearing down efforts - Another fetal risk? Obstet Gyncol 56:39-41, 1980.
14. Ostheimer, GW. Manual of Obstetric Anesthesia, Chapter 4, Churchill Livingstone, New York, 1984.
15. Schellenberg JS.: Uterine activity during lumbar epidural analgesia with bupivacaine. Am J Obstet Gynecol 127:26-31, 1977.
16. Jouppila P, Jouppila R, Hollmen A, et al.: Lumbar epidural analgesia to improve intervillous blood flow during labor in severe preeclampsia. Obstet Gynecol 59:158-161, 1982.

17. Corke BC, Datta S, Ostheimer GW, et al.: Spinal anaesthesia for caesarean section. Anaesthesia 37:658-662, 1982.
18. Hollmen AI, Jouppila R, Koivisto M, et al.: Neurologic activity of infants following anesthesia for cesarean section. Anesthesiology 48:350-356, 1978.
19. Ounsted M, Scott A, Moar V.: Delivery and development: to what extent can one associate cause and effect? J Royal Soc Med 73:786-792, 1980.
20. Klein S. Chapter 6 in Manual of Obstetric Anesthesia, Ostheimer, GW (ed.) Churchill Livingstone, New York, 1984.

TOXEMIA OF PREGNANCY .... YESTERDAY, TODAY AND TOMORROW

GERARD W. OSTHEIMER, M.D.

I. Yesterday (The Past)

Chesley has written an excellent historical review of hypertensive diseases in pregnancy. [1] I would like to quote some interesting historical excerpts from his account:

"In 1897, a veterinarian empirically discovered a cure for parturient paresis in cows, which is now known to be caused by a severe depletion of calcium - he blew air into the teats which stopped lactation. Seeing a similarity between bovine parturient paresis and human eclampsia, Sellheim in 1910, tried the treatment in some of his patients. The breasts were resistant to inflation, so he removed them. His prestige was such that bilateral mastectomy was tried in several clinics but the results, medically and cosmetically, were unsatisfactory."

"At about the same time, postpartum curettage was used in the management of puerperal psychosis, on the hypothesis that some causative substance came from the decidua or retained trophoblast. In 1908, it occurred to Latzko that the eclamptic toxin might have the same source, and he used curettage in the treatment of eclampsia. Several clinics took it up over the next five years, but it disappeared until revived in 1961."

"In 1903, Edebohls proposed renal decapsulation on the hypothesis that eclamptic oliguria and disturbed renal function might depend upon renal edema with compression of the kidney within its unyielding capsule. Sitzenfrey in 1910, found a mortality rate of 39.6% in 58 cases - about twice the rate for eclampsia at that time."

"Zangemeister thought cerebral edema was the cause and in 1911 reported that he had opened the skulls of three living eclamptic women. Wieloch in 1927, used cisternal puncture for the same reason, and drainage of spinal fluid by lumbar puncture was in wide use when I (Chesley) came into the field 42 years ago. Other surgical procedures have included oophorectomy, ventral suspension of the uterus, ureteral catheterization, and implantation of the ureters in the intestine."

"Bizarre as the methods may seem to us, it is important to remember that each was rational in the light of some hypothesis as to the cause and nature of eclampsia. That is more than we can say of our present management, which is empiric, too often symptomatic, and in some respects based upon imitative magic."

"In 1958, Finnerty, Buckholz, and Tuckman reported sensational results with chlorothiazide (Diuril[R]) and acetazolamide (Diamox[R]), which seem to be unconfirmed. They treated sixteen women with severe preeclampsia and all responded with marked decreases in blood pressure and proteinuria; six became normal and were discharged from the hospital before delivery. Finnerty changed his emphasis in all of his later papers, writing that the diuretic drugs prevent the progression of incipient preeclampsia to its hypertensive phase, but are ineffective once the blood pressure has risen."

"Several double-blind studies indicate, however, that the diuretic drugs do not prevent preeclampsia."

"In the recent past, the obstetrician's indiscriminate use of diuretic drugs has not been effective in preventing or treating preeclampsia and in most cases it has been directed against a physiologic change. In general, tampering with physiologic processes is not likely to be beneficial. In addition, there are specific contraindications to the use of diuretic drugs in pregnant women, especially in those with preeclampsia or chronic hypertension."

"The use of diuretic drugs in pregnant women is justified only in the presence of such medical emergencies as cardiac failure, pulmonary edema, or imminent acute renal failure."

"The only rational management (for preeclamsia and eclampsia) is one empirically proved to be effective; the objectives are to prevent convulsions in women with preeclampsia, to stop them in women with eclampsia, and to deliver an undamaged, surviving infant."

"Pritchard[2] has achieved a record unmatched in the history of eclampsia, using only magnesium sulfate, sometimes hydralazine, and delivery. He reported a series of 154 consecutive cases of eclampsia without a maternal death (which he extended to 179 before an accident befell the next patient). In antenatal eclampsia, the uncorrected perinatal loss was 15.4%, with more than half having had no detectable fetal heart beat when treatment was begun; excluding infants weighing less than 1,000g, the perinatal loss was 9.9%. Every infant survived who weighed 1,800g or more and whose fetal heart beat was heard at the beginning of treatment. For comparison, the maternal mortality in eclampsia has ranged up to 70% in the past and is now from 5 to 10% in leading clinics. The perinatal mortality in antenatal eclampsia varies greatly, but a common level is from 20 to 30%."

These fascinating accounts lead us to the current concepts regarding toxemia.

II. Today

A. Definition - Toxemia is the major hypertensive disorder seen in pregnancy. Preeclampsia is the development of hypertension (systolic BP>140 mmHg, diastolic BP>90 mmHg), proteinuria, and/or edema. Eclampsia is the preeclamptic condition associated with grand mal seizures not related to any neurologic disorder. Its cause is still unknown, however, the ultimate problem is decreased uteroplacental blood flow secondary to diminished plasma volume, reduced cardiac output and generalized vasoconstriction.[3] Other problems include: CNS excitability, hepatic dysfunction, renal dysfunction and the possibility of DIC.

B. Predelivery evaluation - History, physical examination and laboratory assessment which includes CBC, electrolytes, BUN, creatinine, creatinine clearance, magnesium, liver enzymes, total protein, albumin, platelets, prothrombin time, partial thromboplastin time, fibrinogen, and fibrin split products.

C. Monitoring techniques available:

1. Blood pressure - cuff acceptable but continuous (I.A. line or automatic device) evaluation preferable.
2. Central venous pressure
3. Electrocardiogram
4. Urine output
5. Deep tendon reflexes and muscle strength
6. Respiratory capability, nerve stimulator
7. Continuous fetal heart rate
8. Continuous uterine contractions
9. Availability of blood gas determinations for fetal scalp capillary blood pH

10. Swan Ganz Catheter (?) - for pulmonary capillary wedge pressure

D. Pharmacologic agents used in the treatment of toxemia:

Drug	Mechanism of Action	Cardiac Output	Renal Blood Flow
1. Magnesium sulfate	CNS depressant mild vasodilation	±	±
2. Hydralazine	direct peripheral vasodilation	↑	0 or ↑
3. Sodium Nitroprusside	direct vasodilator	± ↓	± ↓
4. Nitroglycerin	direct vasodilator	± ↓	± ↓
5. Trimethaphan	ganglionic blockade → vasodilation	↓	↓

E. Vaginal Delivery

    1. Choice of Anesthesia - Continuous lumbar epidural anesthesia is the best choice for pain relief during labor and delivery for the severe preeclamptic if the hematologic studies are normal because intervillous blood flow is improved. (Jouppila et al 1982)[4]

    2. Prerequisites:

      a. Obtain baseline information on all maternal and fetal conditions and medications.

      b. Prehydrate if necessary because of constricted blood volume to raise CVP to 8 to 10cm H_2O. If no CVP line, use 250-1000ml lactated Ringer's solution with 12.5-25g of albumin or equivalent amount of plasmanate.

      c. Avoid aortocaval compression.

      d. Avoid ephedrine if possible.

      e. Immediate availability of cesarean delivery.

F. Cesarean Delivery

    1. Choice of Anesthesia - If a trial of labor has been indicated and an epidural block utilized for analgesia, I would continue with the epidural block if the appropriate level of anesthesia can be obtained. Otherwise, I believe the choice of anesthesia for cesarean delivery is general endotracheal anesthesia.

    2. Prerequisites:

      a. Obtain baseline information on all maternal and fetal conditions and medications.

      b. Prehydrate if necessary because of constricted blood volume to raise CVP to 8 to 10cm H_2O. If no CVP line, use 250-1000ml lactated Ringer's solution with 12.5-25g of albumin or equivalent amount of plasmanate.

      c. Avoid aortocaval compression.

      d. Avoid ephedrine if possible.

      e. Immediate availability of cesarean delivery.

III. Tomorrow

    A. What else? - Prostaglandins!

      Actually the prostaglandin/renin-angiotensin system theory

    B. And finally, Worms!

Lueck et al "discovered" a worm-like organism in patients with toxemia and, subsequently, Aladjem et al induced a toxemia-like syndrome in the pregnant beagle with a concentrate of the organism. We thought we were on the way to a cure for one of the major problems of pregnancy! Fortunately, physicians are also scientists and prefer to duplicate original experiments in their laboratories in order to establish a basis on which to further investigate a problem. Gau et al. did this and the result was the communication "The Worm That Wasn't" (Lancet 1:1160-1161, 1983).

"We were disturbed to read a paper from Lueck et al. stating that preeclampsia, eclampsia, and trophoblastic disease are associated with, and may be caused by, a newly discovered helminth Hydatoxi lualba. This helminth had been observed in smears from circulating blood, trophoblastic tumor tissue, and placentas from toxemic patients. The organism was seen in variable form, as ova, larva, and adult worm.

"Understandably this work has caused interest among obstetricians, pathologists, and the national press. Obstetricians and the press are delighted because any treatable cause of these conditions can only be welcome. As pathologists we were concerned because these helminths have hitherto escaped our attention.

"To investigate these findings we first looked at touch smears of placentas from normal pregnancies, using Lueck's staining technique which involves preliminary exposure of smears to concentrated sulfuric acid. All smears showed organisms identical to those described in the paper. (Fig 6-16). Blood from nonpregnant, predominantly male subjects with no evidence of trophoblastic disease was also examined. All smears were positive. Specimens not subjected to sulfation were always negative.

"Subsequently we looked at transverse sections of these "worms" by both light and electron microscopy and found that they did not have any helminth structure but consisted simply of space surrounded by an anuclear coagulum.

"Clearly these organisms are artifacts produced by the preliminary sulfation in Lueck's staining technique and cannot therefore be responsible for gestational, nor in fact for any other, pathological process."

Further documentation that these organisms are artifacts has been published by Richards et al. from the Centers for Disease Control in Atlanta. (JAMA 250:2970-2972, 1983). These authors could not concentrate these 'helminths' by passing blood through a 12-mm filter although they could demonstrate in stained smears a similar structure to what Lueck et al. found. Their conclusion was that these structures are not helminths but are most likely artifacts.

Therefore, we will not be able to develop a vaccine against toxemia in the near future. In retrospect, I cannot understand why Lueck et al. did not pass their homogenate through a very small filter in order to concentrate the "organism." What fascinates me is that the concentrate from the various preparations was able to produce a toxemia-like state in pregnant beagles. Have investigators isolated the "toxemic factor?"[5]

IV. Summary

Obviously, we don't have an etiology as yet to this multifaceted disease. However, we do have a systematic approach for the utilization of the appropriate analgesia and anesthesia.

References

1. Chesley LC. Management of hypertensive disorders in pregnancy: Then and now. Resident and Staff Physician: 101-105, December 1977.
2. Pritchard JA and Pritchard SA. Standardized treatment of 154 consecutive cases of eclampsia. Am J Obstet Gynecol 123:543-552, 1975
3. Wright JP. Anesthetic considerations in preeclampsia-eclampsia. Anesth Analg 63:590-601, 1983.
4. Jouppila P, Jouppila R, Hollmen A, et al. Lumbar epidural analgesia to improve intervillous blood flow during labor in severe preeclampsia. Obstet Gynecol 59:158-161, 1983.
5. Ostheimer GW.: Yearbook of Anesthesia, p.181-183, Yearbook Medical Publishers, Chicago, 1984.

VOLATILE ANESTHETICS AND THE BRAIN: THE RATIONALE FOR USE IN
NEUROSURGERY
LAWRENCE J. SAIDMAN, M.D.

The introduction of halothane in the mid-1950's represented a
marked advance for anesthesia in the neurosurgical patient.   In
contrast to previously available agents, halothane had the
advantages of being non-irritating, non-flammable, and relatively
insoluble in blood.   In addition, the circulatory effects made it
ideal for induced hypotension.   Its use as an anesthetic for
neurosurgery was great through the 1950's and early 1960's, until
attention was drawn to the fact that intracranial pressure might
rise when halothane was used.[1] This observation was quickly
followed by additional work which substantiated the fact that the
intracranial pressure rose but, more importantly, that it was
especially serious in patients with pre-existing, space-occupying
lesions.[2] The reason for the rise in intracranial pressure was
presumably a consequence of the fact that halothane was shown to
be a potent cerebrovasodilator with the blood flow a function of
anesthetic depth.[3,4] Additional studies at this time revealed
that diethyl ether and cyclopropane were also cerebrovasodilators
and that, like halothane, they both increased cerebral blood flow
out of proportion to cerebral metabolic needs.[5] The final piece
of data regarding the clinical use of halothane in neurosurgical
patients came from the work of Adams, et al., who administered
halothane to patients undergoing craniotomy for tumor or vascular
lesions.[6] Patients receiving the anesthetic were divided into
two groups: those in whom hyperventilation was begun with the
administration of halothane, and those in whom hyperventilation
had occurred prior to the administration of halothane.
Simultaneous hyperventilation resulted in increased intracranial
pressure in 7 out of 21 patients, whereas no patients in the
group in whom prior hyperventilation had occurred had a significant

increase in intracranial pressure. The conclusion was that halothane was capable of increasing cerebrospinal fluid pressure in patients with intracranial disease, but that those increases could be minimized or, in fact, abolished by prior induction of hypocapnea.

Introduction of volatile anesthetics, enflurane and isoflurane, provided hope that perhaps the undesirable vasodilating effects of halothane might be modified and that these agents might be more suitable for anesthesia in patients with space-occupying lesions in the brain. The past few years have seen the publication of a number of papers which support the hope that isoflurane might be a desirable anesthetic for neurosurgical procedures, and I propose to review some of this work which describes cerebrovascular and cerebrometabolic effects of isoflurane on the brain.

Cerebral Blood Flow and Intracranial Pressure

The earliest work looking at the effects of isoflurane on cerebral blood flow was published in 1974 by Murphy.[7] Murphy anesthetized human volunteers at different levels of isoflurane, halothane, and enflurane. With PCO_2 and systemic blood pressure kept at normal levels, halothane was shown to be the most potent cerebrovasodilator, increasing cerebral blood flow almost three-fold at 1 MAC and four-fold at 1½ MAC. In contrast, enflurane approximately doubled cerebral blood flow at 1 MAC, whereas cerebral blood flow was little changed at 1 MAC with isoflurane and approximately doubled at 1½ MAC. Thus isoflurane and, to a lesser extent, enflurane were less potent cerebrovasodilators than halothane. A second human study published in 1981 by Adams repeated the work that had been done earlier with halothane in patients with space-occupying lesions. Repeating the earlier study, patients with brain tumor were divided into two groups: those in whom hyperventilation was begun the same time isoflurane was introduced, and those in whom CO_2 was kept normal. In the isoflurane hypocapnic group, CSF pressure did not increase above awake values following isoflurane administration. In contrast, in the normocapnic patients cerebrospinal fluid pressure consistently increased but could be lowered by establishment of hypocapnia. The conclusion was that the known cerebrovasodilator properties of

isoflurane could be countered effectively by hypocapnia. Furthermore, unlike with halothane, it is not necessary to establish
hypocapnia prior to introducing isoflurane in order to avoid
cerebrospinal fluid pressure increases.

CSF Production

Intracranial pressure can be affected by all intracranial
contents including both cerebral blood volume and the volume of
CSF. Artru has studied the effect of volatile anesthetics on the
rate of formation of cerebrospinal fluid in the dog. He showed
that enflurane significantly increased the rate of cerebrospinal
fluid production and speculated that this might, in part, be
responsible for the late occurring increase in intracranial
pressure observed during prolonged anesthesia with enflurane.[9]
Subsequently he studied the effect of isoflurane on the rate of
CSF production in the dog and found that, with prolonged isoflurane
anesthesia, the rate of CSF production decreased by 8% per hour.
These data suggest that isoflurane causes no significant change in
the rate of CSF production and that an increase in CSF volume does
not occur during prolonged isoflurane anesthesia. Artru goes on
to state that in patients at risk due to increased intracranial
pressure, isoflurane may be preferred to an anesthetic that may
increase intracranial volume such as enflurane or ketamine.[10]
Artru then went on to measure cerebral blood volume and intracranial pressure in dogs anesthetized with isoflurane. He found
that although isoflurane increased cerebral blood volume 9-11%,
ICP increased for only the first 20 minutes. Because halothane or
enflurane increased ICP for greater than 3 hours, Artru states
that isoflurane may be preferred to halothane or enflurane in
patients at risk for increased intracranial pressure.[11]

From these latter experiments it seems that the initial increase
in intracranial pressure and cerebral blood volume caused by
inhalation anesthetics is related to their effects upon the
circulation; that is, cerebrovasodilation. The subsequent return
of intracranial pressure with isoflurane to control probably
reflects both a decrease of CSF volume in response to prior
increase in cerebral blood volume and a subsequent decrease of
cerebral blood volume from peak values as mean arterial pressure

decreases. This is in contrast to prolonged anesthesia with halothane or enflurane which, as mentioned before, increases both ICP and cerebral blood volume for over 3 hours. Halothane and enflurane reportedly increase resistance to reabsorption of cerebrospinal fluid as well as increase in the rate of CSF production. The prolongation of the ICP increase with halothane and enflurane are probably in part a function of this latter effect.

A further indication of the effect of isoflurane on cerebral blood volume comes from a study by Drummond and Todd, who looked at brain surface protrusion with both halothane and isoflurane. They found that brain surface protrusion was considerably greater under halothane anesthesia than isoflurane anesthesia.[12] These findings roughly parallel the effects of these agents on cerebral blood flow and probably reflect the differences in anesthetic-induced changes in cerebral blood volume. The authors go on to say that, if applicable to human anesthesia, these results suggest that in situations during intracranial surgery where administration of a volatile anesthetic is deemed preferable to the use of an additional fixed agent, that isoflurane may be the volatile agent of choice.

Cerebral Metabolic Rate

In a subsequent study designed to further characterize the effects of halothane and isoflurane on cerebral circulation, Todd and Drummond compared the effects of halothane and isoflurane on cerebral blood flow, cerebral vascular resistance, intracranial pressure, and the cerebral metabolic rate for oxygen in cats. They looked at 3 different doses of both drugs (.5, 1.0, and 1.5 MAC) in the presence of 75% nitrous oxide. They found that both agents had similar effects on blood pressure and ICP. However, halothane produced a significant increase in cerebral blood flow with all doses, whereas isoflurane anesthesia caused no significant change in the cerebral blood flow at any level of anesthesia. Both drugs produced dose-related decrease in cerebral vascular resistance, but the changes were greater with halothane. In addition, and most importantly, isoflurane produced greater decreases in $CMRO_2$ than did halothane and also impaired autoregulation less. Clearly, then, isoflurane possesses cerebral vascular properties different than those of halothane, and suggest that isoflurane may come to play an important role in future neuroanesthetic practice.[13] Scheller in a subsequent paper further delineated the difference between halothane and isoflurane. He compared the effects of halothane and isoflurane on cerebral blood flow in rabbits anesthetized with nitrous oxide and morphine at different CO_2 levels.[14] He found that, whereas halothane increases blood flow at all PCO_2 levels studied, isoflurane in fact decreases cerebral blood flow when introduced into hypocapnic rabbits. This is further evidence that isoflurane may be preferable to halothane for use in patients, especially those with reduced intracranial compliance if a volatile agent is considered. Even in animals that had an increase in CO_2, halothane increased cerebral blood flow, whereas isoflurane resulted in no change. An explanation for this is uncertain. It might be due to the metabolic effects of isoflurane, which is a potent inhibitor of cerebral metabolic rate of oxygen to a much greater extent than that of halothane. These latter data, of course, go along with the fact that the electroencephalogram becomes flat much earlier with isoflurane than with halothane, again indicating a greater decrease in $CMRO_2$. Newburg, in a recent paper,[15] investigated the cerebral metabolic effects of isoflurane in animals made hypoxemic or ischemic. In mice breathing 5% oxygen, survival time was increased significantly over control when the animals were breathing 1% or 1.4% isoflurane. Similarly, in dogs the effects of 3% isoflurane on the rate of cerebral ATP and phosphocreatine depletion and lactate accumulation was studied during incomplete global ischemia. In the dogs exposed to isoflurane, the cerebral energy stores were sustained at significantly higher levels than in dogs not breathing isoflurane. Dr. Newburg concluded that circumstances of oxygen deprivation insufficient to abolish cortical electrical activity, isoflurane, like the barbiturates, can provide some cerebral protection, presumably by depressing cortical electrical activity and cerebral metabolism.

The above data all suggest that isoflurane might be a useful

238

volatile anesthetic in patients undergoing neurosurgery, especially those with an intracranial mass. It is less of a cerebrovaso-dilator, does not cause an increase production of CSF, does not impair reabsorption of cerebrospinal fluid, in the presence of low CO_2 may in fact decrease cerebral blood flow, and appears to have a greater depressant effect on the cerebral metabolic rate of oxygen.

In a related paper, Newburg looked at cerebral effects of isoflurane-induced hypotension on dogs. Mean arterial pressure of 50 mmHg or 40 mmHg was associated with a decrease in CBF (60%) and $CMRO_2$ (40%).[16] Most importantly, the cerebral energy state was normal, indicating preservation of aerobic metabolism. This differs from trimethophan, halothane, or nitroprusside hypotension to 40 mmHg where gross alterations in cerebral energy state occurred.[17]

REFERENCES

1. Marx GF, et al: Cerebrospinal fluid pressure during halothane anesthesia. Canadian Anaesthetists Journal 9:239, 1962.
2. Gordon E: The action of drugs on the intracranial contents. Proceedings of the Fourth World Congress of Anesthesiologists in London, 1968: and Jannett WB, et al: The effects of anesthesia on intracranial pressure in patients with space-occupying lesions. Lancet 1:61, 1969.
3. Alexander FC, et al: Cerebrovascular response to $PaCO_2$ during halothane anesthesia in man. J Applied Physiology 19:561, 1964.
4. Wollman H, et al: Cerebral circulation in man during halothane anesthesia: effects of hypocarbia and d-tubocurarine. Anesthesiology 25:180, 1964.
5. Wollman H: Effects of general anesthetics in man on the ratio of cerebral blood flow to cerebral oxygen consumption. In Cerebral Blood Flow, edited by Brock M, et al. page 242, 1969, Apringer Verlag, Berlin.
6. Adams RW, et al: Halothane, hypocapnea, and cerebrospinal fuid pressure in neurosurgery. Anesthesiology 37:510, 1972.
7. Murphy FL, et al: The effects of enflurane, isoflurane, and halothane on the cerebral blood flow and metabolism in man. Abstracts of Scientific Papers, Annual Meeting of the ASA, pp 61-62, 1974.
8. Adams RW, et al: Isoflurane and cerebrospinal fluid pressure in neurosurgical patients. Anesthesiology 54:97, 1981.
9. Artru AA: Relationship between cerebral blood volume and CSF pressure during anesthesia with halothane or enflurane in dogs. Anesthesiology 58:533, 1983.
10. Artru AA: Isoflurane does not increase the rate of CSF production in the dog. Anesthesiology 60:193-197, 1984.

11. Artru AA: Relationship between cerebral blood volume and CSF pressure during anesthesia with isoflurane or fentanyl in dogs. Anesthesiology 60:575, 1984.
12. Drummond JC, et al: Brain surface protrusion during enflurane, halothane, and isoflurane anesthesia in cats. Anesthesiology 59:288, 1983.
13. Todd MM and Drummond JC: Comparison of the cerebrovascular and metabolic effects of halothane and isoflurane in the cat. Anesthesiology 60:276, 1984.
14. Scheller MS, et al: Comparison of the effects of halothane and isoflurane on cerebral blood flow in rabbits anesthetized with nitrous oxide and morphine at different CO_2 levels. Anesthesiology, 1984, in press.
15. Newburg LA and Michenfelder JD: Cerebral protection by isoflurane during hypoxemia or ischemia. Anesthesiology 59:29, 1983.
16. Newburg LA, et al: Systemic and cerebral effects of Isoflurane-induced hypotension on dogs. Anesthesiology 60:541-546, 1984.
17. Michenfelder JD, et al: Canine systemic and cerebral effects of hypotension induced by hemorrhage, trimethophan, halothane or nitroprusside. Anesthesiology 46:188, 1977.

DETECTION OF BRAIN INJURY DURING SURGERY: TODAY AND TOMORROW

LAWRENCE J. SAIDMAN, M.D.

Electroencephalography has historically been restricted to
only a few diagnostic applications. Though not a new procedure
(being used in one form or another for over 75 years), other
than for diagnosing seizure patterns and other focal brain
abnormalities, it has been relegated to a rather obscure place
in modern medicine.

Electrical potentials of the brain of animals were first
noted in 1875 by Caton, and the effects of anesthetics (chloroform
in particular) were first noted by VonMarxow in 1890. Brain waves
were recorded with surface electrodes in 1929, and in the early
30's Gibbs, et al., stated "a practical application might be the
use of the electroencephalogram as a measure of the depth of
anesthesia during surgical operations." The next 20 years were
used to describe the EEG patterns that were associated with the
various anesthetics and more specifically the various depths
associated with any one anesthetic. Though patterns of the
electroencephalogram correlated with anesthetic depth were
described, in fact the EEG did not achieve wide clinical use
in operating rooms. The reasons for this were related to the
following:

1) the type of anesthesia that was being given -- Whereas a
specific EEG pattern could be described for a specific agent at
a specific depth, when combinations of drugs were given, anesthetic
depth identification became impossible.

2) the complexity of and amount of EEG data superimposed upon
the activities of the anesthesiologist -- The amount of and
complexity of data in a conventional EEG recording is too great
for a busy anesthesiologist to pay constant attention to. For
example, a conventional EEG when recorded on paper strip chart

recorders produces data at the rate of over 300 sheets per hour. Obviously the anesthesiologist cannot begin to provide appropriate attention to the EEG. Without being able to continuously monitor the conventional EEG, trends cannot be easily followed. The use of an oscilloscope for electroencephalographic recording is also inadequate for, again, trends cannot be followed and in general the technical quality of oscilloscopic tracing is not sufficient to permit diagnosis of either anesthetic depth or untoward events.

3) development of new agents, new vaporizers, and the description of MAC -- The need for the EEG as a measure of anesthetic depth was minimized by the development of newer and less blood soluble anesthetics such as halothane, fluoroxene, and enflurane as well as vaporizers which, with adequate flow rates, inspired concentration with high flows, low blood solubility, and some knowledge of pharmacokinetics, permitted a reasonably accurate estimation of alveolar concentration and thus brain partial pressure. This, in combination with the description of level of anesthesia in terms of MAC, allowed the anesthesiologist at all times to know the approximate depth of anesthesia as a function of inspired concentration. In my opinion, therefore, our understanding of the interrelationship between MAC, blood solubility, inspired concentration, and fresh gas flows is sufficient to allow a clinically adequate estimation of anesthetic depth without using the EEG.

Use of the EEG in Modern Clinical Anesthesia

The above notwithstanding, I believe there are instances wherein electroencephalographic monitoring is important and results in improved patient care. These are related to surgical procedures and other clinical situations which have in common the possibility of altered or interrupted cerebral perfusion -- to a degree sufficient to cause brain injury and therefore sufficient to cause electroencephalographic changes. Examples of the above are carotid endarterectomy, cardiopulmonary bypass, surgery with associated deliberate hypotension, and long-term barbiturate therapy to control increased intracranial pressure.

Carotid Endarterectomy

Carotid endarterectomy provides perhaps the best example

of how the electroencephalogram can be a useful clinical monitor. It is a procedure wherein cerebral blood flow is interrupted, it has a defined morbidity as a consequence of blood flow interruption, and the technique of surgical management as well as anesthesia can be modified to improve cerebral perfusion if there is evidence of hypoperfusion (reflected as a sudden change in the EEG).

In the absence of the EEG, the most common monitoring technique used for these patients has been to measure stump pressure. This is the pressure in the carotid artery distal to the clamp and is purported to be a measure of perfusion pressure to the brain on the affected side. Conventionally, a pressure of 50 torr is used as an indication that perfusion to the operated side is adequate and that surgery can continue without danger. The difficulty with stump pressure is: 1) it is a single measurement in time and can change during surgery; 2) it does not necessarily indicate that focal problems are occurring; and 3) it does not necessarily indicate adequate cerebral blood flow. For example, it has been shown that there are cases wherein stump pressure over 50 torr is associated with cerebral blood flow of less than 18 ml per 100 g of tissue per minute, and electroencephalographic evidence of hypoperfusion. In contrast, however, the electroencephalogram will, if appropriately used, reflect hypoperfusion and therefore is perhaps a better monitor for adequacy of cerebral perfusion during carotid endarterectomy. If an EEG change is detected, one of a variety of steps can be taken (elevate systemic pressure, insert a shunt, administer barbiturates).

Cardiopulmonary Bypass

Use of the EEG during cardiopulmonary bypass may be of use to detect cerebral hyperperfusion. Preliminary evidence (though not completely agreed upon) demonstrated an EEG abnormality correlated with the severity and duration of hypotension during CPB. As in the case of carotid surgery, increasing perfusion pressure might result in improved blood flow and reduction of EEG signs of hypoperfusion. In the event these maneuvers are not of help, there is some evidence that the use of barbiturates will reduce the damage consequent to clamping of the carotid or hyperperfusion during cardiopulmonary bypass. It obviously must be kept in mind that barbiturates themselves have cardiovascular effects which, when compared with the possible benefit to the brain, may produce an unfavorable cost:benefit ratio. For this reason, in any instance in which barbiturates are considered, factors in addition to their potential saluatory effect on the brain should be taken into consideration.

Barbiturate Coma

Use of high doses of barbiturates to reduce increased intra-cranial pressure has become increasingly popular. In this case EEG monitoring of depth of narcosis is used to indicate when incremental doses of barbiturates are needed.

Requirements for Clinical EEG Monitoring

First, to be reliable and of clinical use, high quality EEG recordings are required. Above all, this requires careful application of electrodes. Whatever technique of application is used, it is important to frequently check the impedence of the leads to avoid artifact as a consequence of a faulty lead.

Second, we feel that multiple leads are required and that bilateral and symmetrical recording is necessary. This is particularly important when looking for focal changes such as those that would be picked up during carotid endarterectomy. The montage we use employs four leads on each side, distributed frontal, occipital, temporal, and mid sagital -- the latter two over the middle cerebral artery.

Third, it is important, particularly when looking for changes as a consequence of perfusion, that the anesthetic level be relatively constant. It would not be of help to be giving frequent doses of barbiturates if one is looking for changes in perfusion consequent to clamping the carotid artery.

Methods of Recording

The conventional EEG has several advantages and disadvantages, some of which were alluded to above. The advantages are the continuous multiple channel detailed recording that ultimately can be reviewed by experts in electroencephalography. The disadvantage of the conventional trace is the amount of data and the difficulty an anesthesiologist has in following trends. Alternative forms of recording which process conventional EEG data into compact records which provide more easy pattern recognition have recently been developed. The first, called the compressed spectral array (CSA) has been in development over the past 8 years and has achieved widespread use in several institutions. This display provides a three-dimensional pictorial representation of electroencephalogram which is essentially a frequency-power histogram with time compressed. Utilizing this form of display, 1 hour's worth of EEG can be compressed into 1 8 x 11 sheet of paper. Thus trends can be followed and an anesthesiologist with an appropriate display device can see changes in the EEG over a long period of time. A typical pattern representing inadequate perfusion shows a decrease in the power of fast activity (>8 hz). A second form of electroencephalographic processing is called density modulated spectral analysis (DSA) which provides a display not very dissimilar from CSA, but which utilizes more conventional equipment. The latter can be plugged into a conventional strip chart recorder. The display is also a frequency power histogram with compressed time such that trends can be easily followed in a way similar to the CSA. Both of these techniques are still in developmental stages, though one or another of them should be available for commercial use in the relatively near future. They probably both will find increased acceptability by anesthesiologists as a consequence of the compressed display and the relatively easy diagnosis of hypoperfusion.

A third example of compressed processed EEG recording is the cerebral function monitor (CFM). The CFM provides a single channel of information, roughly equivalent to integrated microvoltage. The advantages of the CFM are compression of the time domain and weighting of those frequencies most affected by cerebral hypoxia. The drawback of the CFM is all frequency-amplitude information is lost, thus identical recordings result from high-frequency low amplitude and low-frequency high amplitude activity. In addition, record changes may result from frequency or amplitude alone or in combination. In other words, CFM is not sufficiently discriminating.

Sensory Evoked Potentials (EP)

EP are responses of the CNS to sensory stimulation. Normal
EP reflect functioning of various discreet sites in sensory neural
pathways and can be used as a valuable monitor during a variety of
neurosurgical, orthopedic, or vascular procedures.

As with all other monitoring aids, there is a cost:benefit
associated with its use. Costs of EP monitoring include the
requirement for expensive equipment and costly personnel, whereas
the benefits are clearly related to detection of injury before
irreversible damage occurs.

REFERENCES

Carotid Endarterectomy

1. Astrup J, Syman L, Branstron NM, et al: Cortical evoked
    potential and extracellular K^+ and H^+ at critical levels
    of brain ischemia. Stroke 8:51-57, 1977.
2. Boysen G, Engell HS, Pisolese GR, et al: On the critical
    lower level of cerebral blood flow in man, with particular
    reference to carotid surgery. Circulation 6:1023-1025, 1974.
3. Duke PC, Wade JG, Hickey RF, et al: The effects of age on
    baroreceptor reflex function in man. Can Anaesth Soc J 23:
    111-124, 1976.
4. Duke PC, Fownes D, Wade JG: Halothane depresses baroreflex
    control of heart rate in man. Anesthesiology 46:184-187, 1977.
5. Ennix CL, Lawrie GM, et al: Improved results of carotid
    endarterectomy in patients with symptomatic coronary disease:
    an analysis of 1546 consecutive operations. Stroke 10:122,
    1979.
6. Fitch W: Anaesthesia for carotid artery surgery. Br J Anaesth
    48:791-796, 1976.
7. Hoffman JIE, Buckberg GD: The myocardial supply:demand ratio.
    Medical Review. Am J Cardiol 41:327-332, 1978.
8. Hoffman JIE: Determinants and prediction of transmural
    myocardial perfusion. Circulation 58:381-391, 1978.
9. Larson CP Jr: Anesthesia and control of the cerebral
    circulation in extracranial occlusive cerebrovascular disease.
    Diagnosis and Management. Edited by Wylie EJ, Ehrenfeld WK.
    Philadelphia, W.B. Saunders 1970, pp 152-183.
10. Lassen NA, Christensen MS: Physiology of cerebral blood flow.
    Br J Anaesth 48:719-734, 1976.
11. Michenfelder JD, Milde JH, Sundt TM: Cerebral protection by
    barbiturate anesthesia: use after middle cerebral artery
    occlusion in Java monkeys. Arch Neurol 33:345-350, 1976.
12. Smith AL: Barbiturate protection in cerebral hypoxia.
    Anesthesiology 47:285-293, 1977
13. Sublett JW, Seidenberg AB, Hobson RW: Internal carotid artery
    stump pressure during regional anesthesia. Anesthesiology 41:
    505-508, 1974.

14. Sundt TM, Sandok BA, Whisnant JP: Carotid endarterectomy:
    Complications and preoperative assessment of risk. Mayo Clin
    Proc 50:301-306, 1975
15. Wade JG, Larson CP Jr, Hickey RF, et al: Effect of carotid
    endarterectomy on carotid chemoreceptor and baroreceptor
    function in man. N Engl J Med 282:823-829, 1970.

Monitoring the Electroencephalogram

1. Bickford RG, Fleming NI and Billinger TW: Compression of EEG
    data by isometric power spectral plots. Electroencephalography
    and Clinical Neurophysiology, Vol. 31, pp 632-634, 1971.
2. Chiappa KA, Burke SR, Young RR: Results of electroencephalo-
    graphic monitoring during 367 carotid endarterectomies. Stroke
    10:381, 1979.
3. Ehrenfeld WK, Hamilton FN, Larson CP Jr, et al: Effect of CO_2
    and systemic hypertension on downstream cerebral arterial
    pressure during carotid endarterectomy. Surgery, Vol. 67,
    pp 87-96, 1970.
4. Fleming RA and Smith NT: An inexpensive device for analyzing
    and monitoring electroencephalogram. Anesthesiology, Vol. 50,
    pp 456-460, 1979.
5. Gibbs FA, Gibbs EL, and Lennox WG: Effect of electroencephalo-
    gram of certain drugs which influence nervous activity.
    Archives of Internal Medicine, Vol. 60, p 154, 1937.
6. Marshall LF, Shapiro HM, Rauscher LA, and Kaufman NM:
    Pentobarbital therapy for intracranial hypertension and
    metabolic coma. Critical Care Medicine, Vol. 6, pp 1-5, 1978.
7. McKay RD, Sundt TM, et al: Internal carotid artery stump
    pressure and cerebral blood flow during carotid endarterectomy.
    Anesthesiology, Vol. 45, pp 390-399, 1976.
8. Myers RR, Stockard JJ, Fleming NI, et al: The use of unlined
    telephonic computer analysis of the EEG in anesthesia. Br J
    Anaesth, Vol. 45, p 64, 1973.
9. Myers RR, Stockard JJ, and Saidman LJ: Monitoring of cerebral
    perfusion during anesthesia by time compressed fourier
    analysis of the electroencephalogram. Stroke, Vol. 8,
    pp 331-336, 1977.
10. Sadove MS, Becka D, and Gibbs FA: Electroencephalography for
    Anesthesiologists and Surgeons. J.B. Lippincott Co.,
    Philadelphia, 1967.
11. Schwartz MS and Colvin MP, et al: The cerebral function
    monitor. Anesthesiology, Vol. 28, pp 611-618, 1973.
12. Smith NT: Computers in Anesthesia. In Monitoring in
    Anesthesia, edited by Saidman LJ and Smith NT. John Wiley &
    Sons Publishers, New York, 1978.
13. Stockard JJ, Bickford RG, et al: Hypotension-induced changes
    in cerebral function during cardiac surgery. Stroke, Vol. 5,
    pp 730-746, 1974.

Sensory Evoked Potentials

1. Levy WJ, Grundy BL, Smith NT: Monitoring the Electroencephalo-
    gram and Evoked Potentials during Anesthesia. In Monitoring in
    Anesthesia, edited by Saidman LJ and Smith NT, Butterworths
    Publishers, Stoneham, Massachusetts, 1984.

THE NEW MUSCLE RELAXANTS

ROBERT J. FRAGEN, M.D.

Two new nondepolarizing neuromuscular blocking agents have
become available within the last year. Their pharmacology will
be reviewed.

All older skeletal muscle relaxants have one or more side
effects associated with their use and none of them meets the
criteria of an ideal muscle relaxant. Succinylcholine is associated with myalgia, bradycardia, hyperkalemia, increased intraocular and intragastric pressure, tachyphylaxis, non-reversibility
and malignant hyperpyrexia. Tubocurarine and, in high doses,
metocurine can result in hypotension from histamine release and
ganglionic blockade. Gallamine and pancuronium can cause hypertension and tachycardia. All these nondepolarizers have long
durations of action and thus are susceptible to producing prolonged neuromuscular blockade or recurarization. These problems
are exaggerated in patients with ventilatory failure, circulatory
failure, and either hepatic or renal disease. Agents used to
reverse muscle paralysis also have autonomic side effects. The
newer muscle relaxants, atracurium and vecuronium, are virtually
without side effects in clinically useful doses.

Atracurium was introduced by Stenlake in Scotland and developed by Burroughs Wellcome. Atracurium is unique because it
undergoes spontaneous decomposition at body pH and temperature,
Hofmann elimination. A secondary route of metabolism is ester
hydrolysis by other than plasma cholinesterase. Therefore, it
depends on neither hepatic nor renal mechanisms for its elimination. Its elimination half-life is just under 30 minutes. It
comes in a 5 ml ampule containing 10 mg/ml at pH 3.5 and should
be kept refrigerated at $5^{o}C$ to maintain stability. It will
retain 90% of its potency for one month at room temperature in

its acidic solution.

At the ED_{95} dose of 0.2 mg/kg, atracurium causes no side effects. This is usually true for the intubating dose of 0.5 mg/kg, but higher doses can result in histamine release and subsequent cutaneous reactions, hypotension or bronchospasm. A dose of 0.5 mg/kg will provide surgical relaxation for 45-50 minutes and a dose of 0.2 mg/kg for about 20-25 minutes. The recovery index is about 11 minutes. Intubation can be accomplished in about two minutes with a dose of 0.5 mg/kg and increasing the dose will not result in a faster onset time but will only increase the chance of hypotension.

Vecuronium was introduced by Savage in Scotland and the drug was developed by Organon. Vecuronium is pancuronium without a methyl group on the A ring. It is unstable in solution and thus comes in a vial containing 10 mg of crystal vecuronium and a 5 ml ampule of diluent which must be constituted at the time of use. It should then be used within 24 hours. Its elimination half-life is about 100 minutes. Its duration of action is shorter than pancuronium and depends upon redistribution and biliary excretion. Because it is mainly excreted in the bile (80%), it has the same effects in renal diseased patients as in normal patients but has prolonged effects in patients with decreased hepatic blood flow or with hepatic disease.

The ED_{95} is about 0.05 mg/kg and vecuronium will be used clinically in doses that resemble pancuronium doses. The intubating dose will be 0.08-0.1 mg/kg and the maintenance dose will be 0.015 mg/kg. It has been given in a dose of 0.3 mg/kg without causing cardiovascular or other side effects. The onset and duration of vecuronium are shorter than atracurium at ED_{95} doses but when intubating doses are given, both drugs have the same characteristics. A high dose of 0.15 mg/kg will decrease the onset time to about two minutes but increase the duration to about 75 minutes.

Neither drug shows significant accumulation with repeated doses or when given by continuous infusion, but vecuronium is mildly cumulative when the redistribution sites are saturated or the hepatic elimination mechanism cannot keep up with the

dose. Both drugs are easily reversed by the usual doses of
edrophonium, neostigmine or pyridostigmine but edrophonium seems
the most appropriate for these new drugs. With proper monitoring of neuromuscular transmission and proper timing and dosing,
spontaneous return of neuromuscular function is possible without
pharmacological reversal.

Both drugs will be better muscle relaxants for the critically
ill patient and the outpatient because of a duration of action
which is shorter than other nondepolarizing relaxants, the absence of cardiovascular effects, the possibility of spontaneous
recovery, the ease of reversibility and the lessened chance for
recurarization, and the non-dependence on renal mechanisms for
elimination from the body. Neither drug has metabolites with
neuromuscular blocking activity. Both drugs will have the same
drug interactions with antibiotics and succinylcholine as other
nondepolarizers and both should be used with caution in patients
with neuromuscular diseases.

Although neither of these drugs may replace succinylcholine
for rapid sequence induction, a new technique called the 'priming
technique' allows tracheal intubation 60-90 seconds after induction. This technique may be used for any nondepolarizing relaxant.
Described by Dr. Francis Foldes, the first step of the technique
is to give 15% of the intubating dose when the patient enters
the operating room. While waiting the 5-7 minutes for this small
dose to take full effect, the anesthesiologist prepares the patient
for induction, preoxygenates the patient and induces anesthesia.
Two ml of fentanyl should be given with the induction hypnotic.
This is immediately followed by at least 50% of the intubating
dose and intubation can be accomplished in 60-90 seconds. This
is essentially as fast as intubation can be accomplished after
succinylcholine. Doubling the dose of atracurium will increase
the duration of effect by 50% and doubling the dose of vecuronium
will increase its duration of effect by 100%. A guideline for
determining the duration of surgical relaxation in minutes is
to take the dose of vecuronium in micrograms/kg and divide by
two if using a potent inhalation agent and by three if using
a balanced anesthesia technique (i.e. 100 micrograms/kg will

252

provide about 50 minutes of surgical relaxation under enflurane anesthesia).

Because these two drugs wear off rapidly, their effects should be monitored. Also, in those anesthetic techniques which depend upon the tachycardia of the muscle relaxant to offset the brady-cardia of the narcotic (i.e. high dose fentanyl or sufentanil), pancuronium continues to be most appropriate.

Atracurium and vecuronium provide a significant advance in neuromuscular pharmacology because they cause no side effects in clinically useful doses.

REFERENCES

1. Agoston S, Salt P, Newton D et al.: The neuromuscular blocking action of ORG NC45, a new pancuronium derivative in anaesthe-tized patients. Br J Anaesth 52: 535-539, 1980.
2. Basta SJ, Ali HH, Savarese JJ et al.: Clinical pharmacology of atracurium besylate (BW 33A): A new nondepolarizing muscle relaxant. Anesth Analg 61: 723-729, 1982.
3. Fahey MR, Morris RB, Miller RD et al.: Clinical pharmacology of ORG NC45 (Norcuron TM): A new nondepolarizing relaxant. Anesthesiology 55: 6-11, 1981.
4. Fragen RJ, Shanks CA: Neuromuscular recovery after laparo-scopy. Anesth Analg 63: 51-54, 1984.
5. Hughes R, Chapple DJ: The pharmacology of atracurium: A new competitive neuromuscular blocking agent. Br J Anaesth 53: 31-44, 1981.
6. Payne JP, Hughes R: The evaluation of atracurium in anaes-thetized man. Br J Anaesth 53: 45-54, 1981.
7. Savage DS, Sleigh T, Carlyle I: The emergence of ORG NC45... from the pancuronium series. Br J Anaesth 52: 35-39, 1980.
8. Stenlake JB: Ions, cyclic nucleotids, cholinergy; In: Ad-vances in Pharmacology and Therapeutics, ed. by J.B. Stoclet, Oxford, Pergamon Press, 1979.
9. Ward S, Neill EAM, Weatherly BC, Corall IM: Pharmacokinetics of atracurium besylate in healthy patients (after a single I.V. bolus dose). Br J Anaesth 55: 113-118, 1983.

PAIN PATHWAYS AND MECHANISMS

Stephen E.Abram, MD

Until the early 1960's, the perception of pain was
generally considered to be similar to perception of other
sensory modalities, such as touch, pressure and temperature:
activation of a receptor produces volleys of afferent nerve
activity which stimulates ascending neurons in the spinal
cord. Explanations of the wide variation in pain sensibility
among individuals, or in a single individual under varied
circumstances, were not very satisfactory. Pain which
persisted despite cessation of noxious peripheral input was
often felt to be of psychogenic origin. During the last 20
years the concept of straight through transmission of noxious
input has been abandoned. In those two decades a great deal
has been learned about the modulation of nociceptive input in
the peripheral as well as the central nervous system, and
about physical and psychological mechanisms involved in
chronic pain states.

Peripheral Nociceptive Mechanisms

Since the late 1960's, it has become apparent that there
are nerve fibers which are activated only by intense,
tissue-threatening stimuli. The receptors located in skin and
other pain-sensitive tissues have been identified
structurally to be free nerve endings. Afferent axons which
respond exclusively to intense, tissue damaging stimuli,
termed nociceptors, are almost exclusively C or A-delta
fibers, and are classified according to the stimuli which
activate them. There are three major classes. Mechanical
nociceptors respond to intense mechanical stimulation,
although some fibers will respond to thermal stimulation
after sensitization by repeated exposure to heat. These axons
conduct mainly in the A-delta (5-35 m/sec) range.
Mechanothermal nociceptors, also mainly A-delta fibers,
respond to noxious mechanical stimulation, and to noxious
thermal stimulation, even without sensitization. Polymodal
nociceptors are charcterized by their responsiveness to
noxious mechanical or thermal stimuli and to chemical
irritants. The vast majority of polymodal nociceptors are
unmyelinated, and, in humans, all polymodal nociceptors
characterized have been C fibers. Some axons which respond to
temperature changes in the non-noxious range respond to
noxious (>43C) temperatures, but the contribution of these
fibers to the perception of pain is not certain.
Nociceptors have been identified in visceral structures,

such as the heart. It has been proposed, on the other hand, that some types of visceral pain are the result of high-frequency firing of visceral afferents which ordinarily serve homeostatic rather than nociceptive functions. Both C and A-delta nociceptors have been characterized in skeletal muscle. Tooth pulp afferents appear to function exclusively as nociceptors.

Following certain types of peripheral nerve injury, pain may arise without activation of the receptor, or free nerve ending. Wall and Gutnick[3] were able to record spontaneous activity arising from experimentally-induced neuromata. They, along with others, were able to demonstrate increases in spontaneous firing rates following close arterial injection of epinephrine or norepinephrine or following sympathetic stimulation. Dubner postulated that two types of changes occur in growing neuroma sprouts. First, the sprouts acquire an increased number of inward current sodium and calcium channels, which permit spontaneous depolarization. Second, The same areas acquire alpha adrenergic receptors, which, when stimulated, increase spontaneous firing rates.

Another proposed mechanism of pain arising from injured peripheral nerves is the direct activation of nociceptive afferents by sympathetic efferent discharge via artifical synapses, created at the site of nerve damage. While "cross talk" across demyelinated segments may occur, some doubt is cast on this theory by the fact that the phenomenon is a very late consequence of injury, while abnormal afferent impulses begin soon after the damage occurs. In addition, afferent discharges arising from injured nerve segments do not resemble sympathetic outflow patterns.

In addition to spontaneous firing originating from axons, spontaneous activity has been shown to arise from dorsal root ganglia whose peripheral projections have been interrupted. Chronically injured peripheral nerves or nerve roots which do not exhibit spontaneous activity may become sensitive to mild mechanical stimuli, responding with bursts of high frequency discharge and prolonged after-discharge rather than the slower firing and quickly adapting discharge typical of mechanical stimulation of normal afferents[15]. Such phenomena probably explain the acute pain of nerve root compression or peripheral nerve entrapment. Mechanical compression of dorsal root ganglia, as may occur with lateral disc protrusions, may also produce rapid firing and prolonged after discharge.

Certain peripheral reflexes may serve to perpetuate or aggravate painful conditions. Reflex increases in muscle tone, initiated by visceral or somatic pain, may activate muscle and tendon nociceptors. The increase in noxious input initiates further increases in muscle activity, leading to self-sustained motor activity and the development of myofascial pain syndromes. Painful stimulation may also cause reflex increases in sympathetic efferent activity. It has been proposed that prolonged vasoconstriction leads to tissue hypoperfusion and acidosis, changes in extracellular fluid environment, and the release of substances capable of activating or sensitizing nociceptors, such as bradykinin, histamine, 5-hydroxytryptamine and prostaglandins. The subsequent increase in nociceptor activity produces further increases in sympathetic tone, and a so-called "vicious circle" is initiated.

Dorsal Horn Mechanisms

Within the dorsal root, separation of fiber types takes place, with small, thinly myelinated axons becoming arranged laterally, large afferents medially. The small afferents, many of which are nociceptors, enter the dorsal horn directly through the dorsal gray matter, and many synapse with cells in the outermost laminae (I and II), sending a few arborizations into the substantia gelatinosa (laminae II and III). Other fibers penetrate to synapse in deeper laminae or in the dorsal gray commisure. A few C fibers enter the cord via the ventral roots, but their cell bodies are located in the dorsal root ganglia. Large afferents, whose function is primarily transmission of tactile and proprioceptive information, become aggregated in the medial aspect of the dorsal root. They enter the spinal cord medial to the dorsal horn, where they bifurcate, sending a branch upward in the dorsal columns, and another branch laterally, synapsing with cells in laminae IV and V and sending extensive arborizations dorsally into the substantia gelatinosa.

There are three main groups of dorsal horn cells which receive input from primary afferent neurons. Marginal cells in lamina I receive input from unmyelinated and thinly myelinated afferents. They are termed nociceptive specific (NS), respond almost exclusively to noxious stimuli, and send projections to the contralateral thalamus and to more caudal segments of the dorsal horn. Cells in lamina IV, termed low threshold mechanoreceptive (LTM) neurons, receive input from large afferents which respond mainly to tactile stimulation. Many of these neurons send projections through the spinocervical tract to the ipsilateral lateral cervical nucleus. Wide dynamic range (WDR) neurons , located mainly in lamina V, receive both large and small fiber input, and project to the contralateral ventral posterolateral nucleus of the thalamus. WDR neurons fire briefly in response to non-noxious stimuli, but exhibit rapid, prolonged firing following noxious stimulation in their receptive fields.

Cells in the substantia gelatinosa (SG) synapse extensively with dorsal horn neurons which project to the thalamus. Many of these cells exhibit resting discharge in the 5-10 Hz range, and probably exert tonic inhibitory effects on projection neurons (eg WDR neurons). Modulation of the tonic activity of these interneurons is probably effected by descending as well as segmental inputs.

Primary afferent nociceptive neurons activate projection cells via a neurotransmitter, most likely substance P. SG interneurons may inhibit substance P release through

activation of an inhibitory prejunctional receptor.
Enkephalins, short-acting pentapeptide opiates found in
relatively large quantities in the dorsal horn, may serve as
prejunctional inhibitory neurotransmitters. Serotonin and
norepinephrine may act in a similar fashion. Some dorsal horn
projection neurons which respond to noxious stimulation are
suppressed by previous activation of large afferent fibers in
the same segment. This segmental inhibition, which may be
mediated by GABA release, lends support to the original gate
control theory.

Ascending Pathways

The spinothalamic tract (STT) has, historically, been
considered to be the most important pathway for conducting
nociceptive information. It is, indeed, important to pain
perception, but recent information suggests that a number of
other pathways are important as well. The spinothalamic tract
cells of origin lie mainly in lamina I and lamina V. Most
fibers (75%) cross to the contralateral STT. It has been
proposed that fibers projecting to medial thalamic nuclei are
concerned with initiation of the unpleasant, aversive aspects
of pain as well as autonomic responses to pain, while fibers
ending in the posterolateral areas of the thalamus, such as
the ventral posterolateral nucleus (VPL) may be involved with
spatial and temporal characteristics of noxious stimuli.
The spinocervical tract (SCT), located in the dorsolateral
funiculus, ascends without crossing and terminates in the
lateral cervical nucleus, which sends fibers to the
contralateral thalamus. The size of this pathway is variable
in man, and there is probably considerable individual
variation in its role in pain perception.
The dorsal columns probably play a significant role in
transmitting nociceptive information, and appear to be
necessary for normal pain perception. Spinoreticular neurons,
many of which display response characteristics of WDR cells,
project to ipsilateral nuclei in the medullary reticular
formation. These nuclei are known to be important in the
modulation of nociceptive information. Spinomesencephalic
pathways likewise project to areas which are important in
suppressing or augmenting pain perception, such as the
periaqueductal gray. Another possible ascending pain pathway
is the multisynaptic network of short axonal pathways which
crosses and recrosses the midline of the spinal cord.
Reticulodiencephalic fibers, which project from the
medullary reticular formation to the hypothalamus, may, like
the medial aspects of the spinothalamic tract, be important
in initiating affective and autonomic responses. Limbic
forebrain structures are known to be important in initiating
some of the non-discriminative or affective components of
pain. Small surgical lesions in the cingulum bundle have
shown to reduce the distress of intractable pain without
disturbing the patient's ability to perceive and localize
acute pain. The primary somatosensory cortex, which receives

input from the VPL thalamus, may be important for discriminative pain perception.

Descending Control Systems

Evidence for the existence of descending pathways capable of suppressing transmission of nociceptive input came in the early 1970's with the observation that stimulation of the periaqueductal gray (PAG) area of the midbrain, either electrically or by microinjection of morphine, could produce profound analgesia in animals and in man. Anatomic projections from the PAG to the nucleus raphe magnus (NRM) and to medullary reticular formation nuclei were subsequently described. The fact that electrical stimulation of these same medullary nuclei inhibits dorsal horn neurons adds further evidence that they are involved in this descending pain-inhibitory system[10]. A serotonin-containing pathway from the NRM to spinal cord dorsal horn neurons descends via the dorsolateral funiculus[10]. The fibers may activate enkephalin secreting interneurons which suppress firing of projection neurons. There are other, less well defined descending control systems which do not involve endogenous opiate mechanisms. One such pathway contains adrenergic fibers which probably originate in the locus ceruleus[10].

Deafferentation Pain

Following injury to afferent nerve pathways, pain may result from either lack of normal neuronal input or from a reorganization of neuronal structures central to the site of injury. Melzack and Loeser[12] proposed that spontaneous firing of dorsal horn projection cells may occur following destruction of large populations of afferent fibers by rhizotomy, nerve injury or root avulsion. The resultant pain would be perceived in the distribution of the injured nerves. In a similar manner, damage to ascending afferent pathways in the cord, such as the spinothalamic tract, may lead to spontaneous activity in thalamic nuclei, again leading to pain perception. Such a mechanism helps explain the severe pain occasionally felt after cord transsection.

The spontaneous firing of cells in the CNS which occurs after loss of neuronal input is the result of changes at synaptic terminals termed "neuronal plasticity" or "supersensitivity". These changes include: 1) "switching on" of previously ineffective synapses, 2) increased effectiveness of remaining synapses, 3) development of aberrant connections from sprouts of foreign axons, and 4) development of chemical supersensitivity to neurotransmitters released in the vicinity. The result is vigorous activation of pain-projection system neurons by non-noxious stimuli, often from body surface areas not previously within the receptive fields of those cells.

Social and Psychological Factors

Chronic pain may be initiated, or at least aggravated by psychogenic mechanisms. The resultant pain is not simply imagined, and may be as severe and distressing as pain of purely somatogenic origin. Psychological stress may lead to increased release of pain-sensitizing substances such as bradykinin and 5-hydroxytryptamine, precipitating headaches and aggravating many somatogenic conditions. Stress induced muscle hypertonicity causes myofascial pain syndromes and, eventually, muscle shortening, fibrosis and dysfunction. Anxiety produces heightened sympathetic tone which can produce alterations in limb blood flow, changes in extracellular tissue environment and lowered pain thresholds. The descending pain control systems previously described are influenced by cortical functions, and psychopathological conditions may interfere with the tonic inhibitory activity of these pathways.

Depression is a common psychological reaction to pain of somatic origin, and often improves dramatically when the pain improves. However, severe depression may in some cases be the sole cause of pain complaints. The onset of pain can often be traced to a particular event, such as surgery, trauma or an illness, but those events only serve as a trigger for pain behavior and complaints. Symptomatic treatment of such patients is of little help. Following recognition of the problem, treatment should be directed at the depression.

Patients who experience severe pain exhibit a number of expected patterns of behavior. They limit their range of motion and activity, spending much of their time sitting or reclining. They grimace, groan and complain, take medications and visit physicians. If such behavior results in pleasant consequences, such as solicitous attention from a spouse or physician or pleasant psychic effects from analgesics, that behavior becomes reinforced. There is also reinforcement of behavior which enables the patient to avoid unpleasant consequences. Lying in bed may allow the patient to avoid the discomfort caused by physical activity, or to avoid unpleasant social interactions or a disagreeable work situation. Occasionally such operant mechanisms last well beyond the somatic problem which initiated them. In such cases treatment should be directed toward extinguishing the abnormal behavior. Cooperation of the patient's family and physicians is essential.

Secondary gain motives are frequently evident among chronic pain patients. Pain is a symptom which can not be demonstrated or disproven by laboratory studies or physical examination. It is not surprising, therefore, that pain often becomes a defense against intolerable situations or a cause for financial remuneration. In many instances, patients may lose substantial income if their condition is treated satisfactorily, and, whether motivated by conscious or subconscious motives, will not admit to improvement in their condition. On the other hand, they are frequently required by their insurance carriers to continue to seek medical

attention. The health care profession, therefore, is faced
with a substantial number of patients who are preordained
failures. Significantly reduced treatment success rates among
patients injured on the job, receiving financial
compensation, or involved in litigation have been documented.

Another group of patients which plagues the health care
system has been termed the "dissatisfied" pain patients. This
is a fairly homogeneous group, characterized by lack of
response or adverse response to treatment, complicated
medical and surgical history, accident proneness, long pain
duration, inability to work, drug abuse and abnormal
psychological testing. Psychiatric consultation usually
precipitates hostility. These patients should be recognized
by the physician in order to isolate them from other
patients, as they are often disruptive to group programs, and
to avoid continued fruitless therapeutic intervention.

REFERENCES

1. Dubner R, Bennett GJ: Spinal and trigeminal mechanisms of nociception. Ann Rev Neurosci 1983;6:381-418.

2. Yaksh TL, Hammond DL: Peripheral and central substrates involved in the rostrad transmission of nociceptive information. Pain 1982;13:1-85

3. Wall PD, Gutnick M: Ongoing activity in peripheral nerves: the physiology and pharmacology of impulses originating from a neuroma. Exp Neurol 1974;43:580-593.

4. Devor M, Janig W: Activation of myelinated afferents ending in neuroma by stimulation of the sympathetic supply in the rat. Neurosci Lett 1981;24:43-47.

5. Devor M: Nerve pathophysiology and mechanisms of pain in causalgia. J Auton N Syst 1983;7:371-385.

6. Murphy RW: Nerve roots and spinal nerves in degenerative disc disease. Clin Orthop 1977;129:46-60.

7. Zimmerman M: Peripheral and central nervous mechanisms of nociception, pain and pain therapy: facts and hypotheses. In Bonica JJ et al (eds) Advances in Pain Research and Therapy vol 3. New York, Raven Press, 1979. pp3-32.

8. Willis WD, Coggeshall RE: Sensory Mechanisms of the Spinal Cord. New York, Plenum, 1978.

9. Casey KL: Neural mechanisms of pain: an overview. Acta Anaes Scand 1982; suppl 74:13-20.

10. Basbaum AI, Fields HL: Endogenous pain control mechanisms: review and hypothesis. Ann Neurol 1978;4:451-462.

11. Duggan AW: Transmitters involved in central processing of nociceptive information. Anaesth Intens Care 1982;10:133-138.

12. Melzack R, Loeser JD: Phantom body pain in paraplegics: Evidence for a central "pain generating mechanism" for pain. Pain 1978;4:195-210.

13. Sternbach RA: Psychological factors in pain. In Bonica JJ, Albe-Fessard D (eds) Advances in Pain Research and Therapy, vol1. New York, Raven Press, 1976. pp 293-299.

14. Fordyce WE: Learning processes in pain. In Sternbach RA (ed) The Psychology of Pain. New York, Raven Press, 1978. pp 49-72.

15. Pace BL: Psychophysiology of pain: diagnostic and therapeutic implications. J Fam Pract 1977;5:553-557.

NON-CHEMICAL METHODS OF MANAGING PAIN

STEPHEN E. ABRAM, MD

INTRODUCTION
    The Anesthesiologist's role in pain management has, historically, been confined mainly to several areas: 1.) nerve block therapy of acute and chronic pain, 2.) pharmacologic and regional anesthetic management of postoperative and cancer pain. As they have increased their involvement in pain clinic settings, it has become increasingly obvious to many anesthesiologists that neither nerve blocks nor conventional analgesic agents are appropriate for the majority of patients with chronic pain of non-malignant origin. Indeed, the use of conventional medical techniques, such as blocks, surgery and prescription drugs is likely to reinforce illness behavior among chronic pain patients, and many of the drugs which are useful for acute pain produce tolerance and, perhaps, suppression of intrinsic pain suppression mechanisms when used long-term. There has been a great deal of interest, therefore, in non-pharmacologic techniques. Some of these techniques have the added advantage of being self-administered, implying an increased role of the patient in his/her own recovery. This presentation will discuss several non-chemical and, for the most part, non-invasive techniques which are in use or are being evaluated for chronic pain management.

TRANSCUTANEOUS ELECTRICAL NERVE STIMULATION (TENS)
    TENS was first introduced in the early 1970's as a prognostic procedure to predict the efficacy of implanted peripheral nerve stimulators. It soon became apparent that patients could maintain analgesia through the repeated use of the device. Most units deliver a non-symmetrical biphasic pulse wave. The earlier devices employed frequencies of 20 to 100 Hz, and current amplitude was kept in a range which was non-painful and which did not produce muscle contraction. More recently, capability has been added for low frequency (2-4 Hz) high intensity (producing muscle contraction and, occasionally some discomfort) stimulation. This so-called "acupuncture-like" stimulation probably acts by a different mechanism than high frequency TENS, and has been postulated to release endogenous opiates.
    Several possible mechanisms of action have been proposed for the analgesia induced by TENS. Selective stimulation of large afferent fibers, which have been shown to have a lower threshold to activation by repetitive electrical stimulation, has been postulated to act through a dorsal horn gating

mechanism. High frequency stimulation has been shown to selectively block activity of small afferents, particularly C-fibers, in peripheral nerves. Low frequency TENS, as previously mentioned, may cause the release or activation of endogenous opiates or other pain-modulating substances.

TENS has been employed successfully for both acute and chronic pain states. It is often of benefit for post-operative pain, allowing decreased analgesic use and improved mobility. Likewise, benefit to patients with post-traumatic pain, such as rib fracture, has been documented. Pain from uterine contractions during the first stage of labor is reduced in some patients, but the technique suffers from the disadvantage that the electric current interferes with fetal monitoring devices. Most discussions of TENS for control of chronic pain indicate a 20 t0 30% long term success rate. While initial response is much higher, many patients do not continue to benefit after the first few weeks. A wide variety of pain problems, including myofascial pain, sympathetic dystrophy, and deafferentation syndromes (post-herpetic neuralgia, phantom limb pain, nerve root compression) have been successfully treated. The technique may also benefit some cancer pain patients.

ACUPUNCTURE

There are some reasonably well documented studies which attest to the effectiveness of acupuncture in humans as well as in animal models. While there is little doubt that the technique has physiologic effects, there is growing scepticism that the traditional scheme of acupuncture points is as important as originally postulated. Indeed, there are some recent studies that suggest that stimulation of non-acupuncture points is as effective as stimulation of "appropriate" acupuncture points, and that stimulation on the surface of the skin is as effective as stimulation by acupuncture needle electrodes. There seem to be two reproducible facts regarding low-frequency or acupuncture-like stimulation, which are true whether needles or surface electrodes are used: 1.) stimulation outside the segmental pain distribution produces some analgesia, and 2.) stimulation within the segmental distribution of pain produces better analgesia than stimulation outside the involved segment.

Based on the controlled, reproducible data which now exists, it would appear that low frequency, high intensity stimulation is best delivered via surface electrodes, utilizing a portable device which the patient can operate at home. There seems to be little advantage to traditional needle acupuncture other than the financial benefit to the acupuncturist.

Auriculotherapy is a form of acupuncture which is based on a belief that there is a representation of all parts of the body on the ear, and that stimulation of the appropriate point on the ear will relive pain in that part of the body represented by that point. A recent controlled study by

Melzack failed to show any analgesic effect by the technique.

IMPLANTED NEURAL STIMULATION DEVICES
Direct stimulation of peripheral nerves or of certain
areas in the spinal cord or brain may produce effective
analgesia in patients who are unresponsive to TENS or
acupuncture. In general, these techniques require surgical
implantation of electrodes and electrical stimulators,
although, in some instances, electrodes can be placed
percutaneously, as in the case of epidural stimulating
devices. Peripheral nerve stimulators are usually placed
surgically under direct vision. They are usually employed for
peripheral neuralgias which have been unresponsive to nerve
blocks, TENS, or surgical procedures such as neurolysis or
neurectomy.
Stimulation of the spinal cord was originally done with
so-called dorsal column stimulators. Such devices were placed
via laminectomy, and were felt to act by stimulation of
pathways lying in the dorsal aspect of the cord which carry
input primarily from large afferent neurons. It later became
apparent that other areas of the cord were involved in the
antinociceptive action of the technique, and combinations of
anterior and posterior electrodes were employed, with
somewhat better success. Systems have recently been developed
for percutaneous placement of dorsal stimulating electrodes
into the epidural space which can be tunnelled to a
subcutaneous stimulator. Although the technique avoids a
laminectomy, there is a higher failure rate caused by
improper placement or migration of the electrodes. A recent
long term followup of patients with dorsal column stimulators
by Long demonstrtes significant relief in 1/3 of patients,
with some failures resulting from hardware problems, and
others from a decline in efficacy despite normal function of
the device.
Nashold has employed a modified technique for spinal cord
stimulation in patients with lumbar radiculopathy, placing
one electrode epidurally and the other into the neural
foramen of the involved nerve root. Larson and Abram have
employed a similar technique, using two percutaneously placed
lumbar paravertebral electrodes.
Stimulation of the periaqueductal gray (PAG) area of the
midbrain was shown, in the late 1970's to produce profound
analgesia in animals and in humans with intractable pain. The
analgesia so produced was found to be naloxone reversiable,
suggesting mediation by activation or release of endogenous
opiates. The technique had several drawbacks, including
visual disturbance during stimulation, and the rapid
development of tolerance. More recently, other areas, such as
the periventricular gray and some areas of the reticular
formation, have been stimulated with good results and fewer
side effects.

OTHER PHYSICAL MODALITIES
A variety of physical forms of therapy, some of which have

proven effectiveness for acute pain, have been applied to
patients with chronic pain problems. Diathermy involves
selective heating of deep tissues. Ultrasound diathermy has
become popular with physical therapists because of its
superior tissue penetration, short treatment time (3-10 min)
high differential effect between fat and muscle, and safe use
over metal implants. It appears to have at least short term
benefit for myofascial pain.

The application of cold to the skin surface, either by the
application of ice or by spraying with volatile liquid (ethyl
chloride, fluorimethane) has been shown clinically and
experimentally to produce transient analgesia within the
segment stimulated. Such applications rarely produce lasting
benefit when used alone, but are helpful in providing
transient analgesia to permit stretching and range of motion
exercises to be carried out. Vibration likewise has been
shown to reduce painful sensation within the stimulated
dermatome. Both cold and vibration are thought to produce
analgesia through activation of non-nociceptive afferents
which are capable of suppressing pain-projection neurons in
the dorsal horn.

Manipulation therapy is based on the assumption that many
pain problems stem from malalignment or subluxation of the
spinal column. Numerous studies fail to document any
long-term benefit from manipulation. Traction, like
manipulation, has been used frequently for both acute and
chronic low back pain. The theory that traction works by
reducing pressure on the disc is ill-founded, since 50-100
lbs, rather than the usual 10-15, is needed to produce such
an effect. Traction generally has not been shown to have more
than a placebo effect, but may have the benefit of enforcing
bedrest when immobilization is truly indicated. Braces,
collars and corsets are widely prescribed, but, for chronic
pain problems, are usually of benefit only for the orthopedic
supply dealers. Long term use of such devices tends to weaken
supporting muscles, which eventually shorten and fibrose, and
to cause limitation of motion.

Laser biostimulation is a relatively new modality
utilizing low-energy helium-neon laser skin stimulation. Very
little literature on the subject has reached the scientific
press, possibility because of its lack of efficacy. One
recent study reports excellent short term results in only 26%
of patients (less than one would expect from placebo). No
long term data have been published.

PSYCHOTHERAPEUTIC TECHNIQUES

EMG biofeedback and relaxation training have attained
widespread use in the management of chronic pain. The
rationale for their use is based on the assumption that many
chronic pain problems, particularly headache, are related to
abnormally increased muscle tension. There seems to be some
efficacy in reducing muscle tone by these modalities, but the
effectiveness of these techniques in suppressing chronic pain
has not been conclusively demonstrated. They may be useful as

a part of a multidimensional pain program, however.

Many patients, through positive reinforcement of so-called "pain behaviors", eg continued verbal complaints, drug use, seeking medical attention, limitation of activity, obtain positive reinforcement (financial reward, attention) or avoid negative reinforcement (unpleasant work or social situations, family responsibilities). Operant tratment programs seek to eliminate pain behavior through the elimination of such reinforcers in the patient's environment. Operant conditioning does appear to increase activity levels and to decrease medication use. Cognitive therapy, which attempts to correct faulty or distorted beliefs regarding pain (eg the belief that all pain signifies tissue pathology) or expectations of treatment, has been shown to decrease the number of pain complaints. Hypnosis can be regarded as an extension of cognitive treatment.

PATIENT CONTROLLED ANALGESIA VS CONVENTIONAL POSTOPERATIVE PAIN MANAGEMENT

Bradford D. Hare, M.D., Ph.D.

Introduction

Post-operative pain is a major concern to patients undergoing surgery. Unfortunately many patients find their pain is inadequately treated, partially because of individual variability in analgesic requirements, but more importantly, because too little analgesic is prescribed too seldom or on a PRN schedule. The physician's fear of narcotic side effects, primarily respiratory depression and physical dependence, are largely responsible for the ineffective use of analgesics. Oftentimes, analgesics are prescribed with flexibility in both dose and schedule, but under these circumstances, because of initial underprescribing and nursing fear of overmedication, minimum doses are given. As a result the patient has less than adequate pain relief and little control in this situation, and, therefore, fears and anxiety compound the problem.

Much emphasis recently has been placed on the discovery and introduction of new analgesics agents. Whereas the agents we have available to us at present are not perfect or free from side effects and other problems, with more efficient and effect use of these agents, much better pain relief could be achieved. Patient controlled analgesia, which offers patient control of dosing parameters, appears to offer the potential to overcome many of these basic problems.

Basics of Post-operative Pain Control

Considerable research has been devoted to the identification of important factors for control of post-operative pain. It has become apparent from this research there are many problems that need to be overcome, including huge individual variation in post-op pain medication requirements, different analgesic requirements for different surgical procedures, and the necessity for compensation for changing medication requirements. Tamsen, et al, (9) have demonstrated that with optimal post-op analgesic administration, a 3-4 fold difference in serum levels of analgesic were required for adequate relief. Other studies (2,6) would suggest that this variability may even be greater, perhaps 10-30 fold. Under these circumstances, achieving and maintaining appropriate blood levels obviously is a difficult problem. Commonly, the nurse is supplied with orders allowing considerable flexibility in the amount and schedule of administered narcotics, and it is left to her/his discretion to give medications when appropriate. The medications are ordered on a PRN schedule which leads to delays, and anxiety concerning pain medications grows within the patient. This in turn appears to actually increase the amount of pain medication required, and PRN administration of narcotics is an inefficient and ineffective attempt at post-op pain relief.

Ideally, the patient should have consistent pain relief without side effects such as sedation, nausea, or respiratory depression. If relatively constant, appropriate blood levels of analgesic agent could be achieved with balance between pain relief and side effects, the relief would be optimal. This is really quite difficult with intermittent narcotic doses. Intermuscular injections can allow reasonable pain relief, but the blood levels vary quite widely leading to inconsistent pain relief and occurrence of side effects, particularly at the time of peak effect. On the other hand, techniques such as constant I.V. infusion allow constant blood levels of analgesia, but the flexibility in compensating for changes in analgesic needs and the tendency for accumulation of excess analgesic with time are major drawbacks to this technique.

At the same time, the I.V. route certainly does have attractive aspects. The medication achieves peak effect in a very short time, and the onset of pain relief is rapid. Since I.V. medications have a shorter duration, more exact pain control, with changing needs, can be achieved and maintained. If side effects occur, restriction of the medication for a short period of time will reduce these side effects. These rapids shifts, though, can be a drawback to I.V. analgesia since this would require frequent nursing observation and changes in medication administration. Patient controlled analgesia, on the other hand, would allow the patient to regulate I.V. medication, thus eliminating the need for the nurse in the immediate feedback loop for medication control (4).

Patient Controlled Analgesia (PCA)

Patient controlled analgesia is a technique of analgesic administration with which the patient can self-administer incremental doses of intravenous analgesic for the control of pain. Whereas the dose and maximum frequency are prescribed by the physician, the actual administration is triggered by the patient as needed for pain. Since only a maximum safe dose is dictated, the patient may self-administer narcotics up to this level as needed to achieve the ideal balance between analgesia and analgesic side effects. With the rapid onset of I.V. medication, the patient can achieve very tight control of his pain. In addition to the actual pharmacologic effects of medication, patient controlled analgesia appears to reduce the anxiety, which in itself often reduces the effectiveness of analgesics when administered by the more conventional PRN means or when the patient is dependent on the nurse for medication. There is likely a placebo effect (7) to enhance the pharmacologic effect particularly if the visual or auditory response of the equipment is the same for an injection or an attempt during the lockout period.

The equipment (Harvard Syringe Pump, C. R. Bard, Inc.) which has only recently become commercially available, consists of a computer controlled syringe pump. Dose and maximum frequency of injection can be programmed and data regarding hourly doses and attempts can be retrieved. A standard 50 cc syringe serves as the container for the narcotic. The patient triggers this pump as needed for pain and at this time would receive a small dose of I.V. narcotic, most commonly morphine. Generally, the dose of morphine is 1-3 mg, and the maximum frequency ranges from 6 to 15 minutes. With morphine it would seem reasonable to use the longer lock-out period since peak brain levels with I.V. administration are not achieved until approximately 12 minutes after administration. Even though the patient, in fact, has control over the actual administration of the narcotics, the safety parameters effectively prevent the occurrence of anticipated side effects such as respiratory depression. As will be discussed later, respiratory depression, sedation, nausea, and other side effects with narcotics appear to be less with patient controlled analgesia.

Comparison of Patient Controlled Analgesia With Other Methods of Parenteral Analgesic Administration

Numerous studies have reported on the usages and benefits of patient controlled analgesia. These have recently been reviewed (5). A comparison of one means of post-operative pain control to another must include considerations of a number of parameters. These would include: (1) pain relief, (2) side effects, (3) amount of medication used, (4) patient preference, (5) post-op recovery, (6) cost advantage, (7) method specific disadvantages or contraindications. The following discussion will revolve around these parameters.

Adequacy of pain relief is probably the most important measure in comparing one method of post-operative pain control to another. In theory, patient controlled analgesia should be superior since patients can titrate medication against pain and maintain uniform pain relief. Studies by Bennett (2) have found PCA to offer superior pain relief over PRN medication both in quantity and uniformity. We recently completed a study comparing morphine by PCA to regularly scheduled I.M. morphine rather than a comparison to inferior PRN medication as done by Bennett. In this study we fully expected I.M. morphine on a regular schedule to compare more favorably to patient controlled analgesia, and we, in fact, found consistently less pain with patient controlled analgesia but no statistical difference between these two methods.

Side effects of analgesics often limit the dose of medication that can be used, and pain relief may be compromised. Optimal administration of analgesics should increase analgesia while the side effects would plateau or decrease. The narcotic analgesics have inherent a number of potential side effects, the most serious of which is respiratory depression. In most studies with patient controlled analgesia, this has not been a major problem, particularly when reasonable observation and patient instruction have occurred beforehand, although there have been reported problems under certain circumstances such as use in hypovolemic patients (8). Less drastic but more frequent problems are those of nausea and sedation. Occurrence of these problems not only leave the patient uncomfortable in the case of nausea, but with sedation the post-operative ambulation and respiratory function of the patient may be reduced, leading to potential serious consequences. Again, patient controlled analgesia would appear to offer an advantage since lower maximum serum analgesic concentrations would be expected. In our study nausea was significantly less with PCA by both patient/nursing report and by the amount of anti-nausea medication used. This has been reported consistently in other studies (2). On the other hand, sedation, which has been reported less with patient controlled analgesia (2), was not found by observation or statistics to be less with PCA in our study. In both groups the sedation level was rated acceptable. As we anticipated, the more optimal I.M. medication on regular schedule (as compared to PRN) reduced the advantage in side effects of PCA over IM administration.

The amount of medication used could be an indicator of potential side effects, but it is only important if side effects do in fact increase with a higher dose. Other studies (26) have shown less medication is used with patient controlled analgesia. Our study contrasts with these results since we found a consistently greater, but not a statistically significant different morphine consumption with PCA. At the same time, the side effects were not increased but reduced, a finding which would reduce the negative implications of this observation.

Patient preference, while difficult to quantitate, is an important consideration within certain practical limits. The patients in our study and as reported in other studies consistently seem to prefer PCA over I.M. medications. Some reasons are obvious, such as less discomfort with IV drug administration. On the other hand, a factor less easy to identify and quantitate is that of the patient's control. Patients feel that they have greater control over their pain, which likely reduces anxiety, improves their pain control, and promotes placebo effect over and above the pharmacologic effect.

Post-operative recovery parameters such as respiratory function and ambulation are extremely important and are related to the balance between analgesia and undesirable side effects with the analgesics, such as over sedation and respiratory depression. Studies by Bennett (1,3) would suggest that respiratory function and activity are, in fact, improved with PCA compared to more conventional analgesic administration. Although we did not specifically document improvement in these parameters, our nursing staff subjectly felt that patient controlled analgesia offered better recovery in both respiratory function and ambulation.

Cost advantage with today's concern for cost effectiveness is an important point of comparison. At this time a cost comparison of PCA to other types of post-operative pain relief is not available. General considerations including nursing and pharmacy costs would suggest little difference from conventional techniques. The cost of the PCA equipment must be considered. With reduced side effects and improved post-op parameters in ambulation and respiratory function, shorter hospital stay would be expected with PCA, a factor that could provide significant cost savings.

Although there are a number of clear-cut advantages to patient controlled analgesia, as listed above, this technique is not without some limitations and disadvantages. Patients must have intravenous line in place; the patient must be able and willing to participate in his own care and must be adequately instructed as to this participation. Respiratory depression, while not a common problem, can occur particularly in hypovolemic patients (8). This technique is not recommended for patients with a history of drug abuse since it would be anticipated that the patient might have difficulty separating out medication for pain treatment versus medication for recreational purposes. On the other hand, for patients who have narcotic tolerance due to prolonged narcotic use in post-trauma or in cancer, this could be an ideal means for compensating for increased analgesic requirements if the patient undergoes further surgery and has a need for increased pain medication.

Conclusion

Patient controlled analgesia is a unique method of analgesic administration which appears superior to other means of conventional pain management. The side effects occurring with patient controlled analgesia appear to be less frequent and less severe than those with analgesics given by other parenteral means. The patients clearly prefer this method over I.M. injections and feel that they have more control over their pain. Even though there are some method specific disadvantages, patient controlled analgesia appears to be a superior method of post-operative pain control which makes optimal use of commonly available narcotic analgesics.

REFERENCES

1. Bennett RL, Batenhorst RL, Foster TS, Griffen WO, Wright BD: Postoperative pulmonary function with patient-controlled analgesia (abstract). Anesth Analg 61:171, 1982.
2. Bennett RL, Griffen WO: Patient-controlled analgesia. Contemporary Surgery 23:75-89, 1983.
3. Bennett RL, Batenhorst RL, Graves D, Foster TS, Bell RM, Bivins B, Griffen WO, Wright BD: Patient-controlled analgesia: A new concept of postoperative pain relief. Annals of Surgery 195:700-705,1982.
4. Dahlstrom B, Tamsen A, Paalzow L, Hartvig P: Patient-controlled analgesic therapy, part IV: Pharmacokinetics and analgesic plasma concentrations of morphine. Clinical Pharmacokinetics 7:266-279, 1982.
5. Graves DA, Foster TS, Batenhorst RL, Bennett RL, Baumann T: Patient-controlled analgesia. Ann Intern Med (June, 1983).
6. Keeri-Szanto M: "Demand analgesia" from Trends in Intravenous Anesthesia. Eds: Aldrete JA, Stanley TH. Year Book Medical Publishers, Chicago, 1980.
7. Keeri-Szanto M: Drugs or drugs: What relieves postoperative pain? Pain 6:217-230, 1979.
8. Tamsen A, Hartvig P, Fagerlund C, Dahlstrom B, Bondesson U: Patient-controlled analgesic therapy: Clinical experience. Acta Anaesth Scand 74:157-160, 1982e.
9. Tamsen A, Sakurada T, Wahlstrom A, Terenius L, Hartvig P: Postoperative demand for analgesics in relation to individual levels of endorphins and substance P in cerebrospinal fluid. Pain 13:171-183, 1982d.

TOXICITY OF LOCAL ANESTHETICS

A.P. WINNIE

SYSTEMIC TOXICITY

Local anesthetic agents are employed to provide regional anesthesia by reversibly blocking nerve conduction in peripheral nerves, an effect that is accomplished by the ability of local anesthetic agents to inhibit the excitation-conduction process in the cell membrane of nerve tissue. However, if the concentration of local anesthetic agents is allowed to increase significantly above that concentration required to block conduction and peripheral nerves, all excitable membranes such as those in the central nervous system, and in cardiac and vascular smooth muscle can be affected similarly. Ordinarily, when doses of local anesthetic appropriate for a particular block in a particular patient are properly injected perineurally, signs of systemic toxicity·are rare. However, either improper placement of an appropriate dose of local anesthetic (into a blood vessel) or appropriate placement of an excessive dose of local anesthetic can result in blood and tissue levels that will produce serious systemic effects.

The central nervous system is particularly susceptible to the systemic effects of local anesthetic agents, and shows signs of progressive stimulation followed by progressive depression. If the blood level of local anesthetic rises slowly, has after a properly placed but excessive dose of local anesthetic, the signs of central nervous system toxicity progress slowly and, if inadequately treated, culminate in generalized convulsions of a tonic-clonic nature. On the other hand, if a sufficiently large dose of a local anesthetic is administered accidentally intravenously, the early signs of central nervous system excitation may be missed, seizure activity begins almost immediately, and may rapidly be replaced by a state of generalized central nervous system depression, which includes progression to respiratory depression and even arrest. The mechanism by which local anesthetics produce their excitatory effect on the brain is believed to involve a selective blockade of inhibitory pathways in the cerebral cortex, allowing facilitatory neurons to function unopposed, resulting in an increase in excitatory activity leading to convulsions. Larger doses of local anesthetics simply inhibit both inhibitory and facilitatory pathways, resulting ultimately in a generalized state of central nervous system depression. The central nervous system toxicity of a local anesthetic appears to be related in general to the intrinsic anesthetic potency of the agent, so the relative CNS toxicity of bupivacaine, etidocaine, and lidocaine is approximately $4:2:1$ which is similar to the relative potency of these agents for the production of epidural anesthesia in man. The acid-base status of a patient has an important impact on the central nervous system toxicity of the local anesthetic, and animal work indicates that there is an inverse relationship between the PCO_2 and the convulsive threshold. This important relationship between PCO_2 and the effect of local anesthetics on the central nervous system results from the fact that an elevation of PCO_2 will enhance cerebral blood flow so the more anesthetic agent is delivered to the brain; and in addition, diffusion of CO_2 across the nerve membrane may result in a fall in intracellular pH, which will favor ionic trapping of local anesthetics within the nerve cells.

As a rule, the cardiovascular system appears to be more resistant to the effects of local anesthetic agents than the central nervous system, as evidenced by animal studies which indicate that doses which cause significant cardiovascular depression are approximately three times higher than those which produce convulsions. The toxic effects of local anesthetics on the heart are manifest by a progressive sequential depression of the pacemaker and the conduction system of the heart with increasing blood levels, and a similar progressive depression of the mechanical activity of the heart muscle itself. Thus, electrophysiologic studies indicate that as the dose and blood levels of local anesthetic are increased, a prolongation of conduction time through the various parts of the heart occurs, and extremely high concentrations of local anesthetics will ultimately depress spontaneous pacemaker activity in the sinus node and atrial ventricular node. Similarly, animal studies indicate that all local anesthetics exert a dose-dependent negative inotropic action which correlates with their local anesthetic activity.

While it is true that local anesthetic agents have a biphasic action on the smooth muscle of peripheral blood vessels, toxic levels of local anesthetics uniformly produce vasodilatation, and when this action is superimposed on the negative inotropic effect of the local anesthetics on the heart, the combined effect will be cardiovascular collapse and ultimately cardiac arrest.

While the degree of cardiovascular depression produced by local anesthetic agents is usually directly related to the potency of the individual agents, recently there is evidence that the more potent, highly lipid soluble, and highly protein-bound local anesthetic agents may be relatively more cardiotoxic than the less potent, less lipid soluble, and less protein-bound local anesthetics. Cases have been reported in which bupivacaine and etidocaine were associated with rapid and profound cardiovascular depression and/or severe cardiac arrhythmias following accidental intravascular injection, sequelae which in most cases appeared to be particularly resistant to the usual therapeutic measures. Most of the reports of sudden cardiovascular collapse and death involve the use of bupivacaine 0.75% in obstetrical patients, and as a result, the use of this concentration of bupivacaine for epidural anesthesia in obstetrics is no longer recommended in the United States. The etiology of these un-toward responses is still not known, and to date animal studies have produced puzzling and conflicting data. However, in view of the potential cardiotoxicity of bupivacaine, every effort must be made to avoid an accidental intravascular injection with this drug, and the use of a test dose of local anesthetic with epinephrine is strongly recommended; and in addition slow injection or fractional doses should be utilized when per-forming techniques requiring large volumes of local anesthetic agent.

It has already been mentioned that changes in acid-base status will alter the central nervous system toxicity of local anesthetics, and the same is true with cardiovascular toxicity. Thus hypercarbia and acidosis (and hypoxia) will tend to increase the cardiodepressant effects of local anesthetics. Since hypercarbia, acidosis, and hypoxia can occur very rapidly following seizure activity, the cardiovascular depression observed with the more potent agents such as bupivacaine may be related in part to the severe acid-base changes that occur following the administration of toxic doses of these agents.

LOCAL (NEURO) TOXICITY

Used in clinical concentrations, the potential of local anesthetic agents to cause localized nerve damage is extremely low. It would seem that the spinal cord and spinal nerve roots might be more vulnerable

when the local anesthetic is injected intrathecally, since they lack a connective tissue sheath. However epidemiological studies on spinal anesthesia have repeatedly indicated that neurotoxicity is not a major problem. Recently, reports of prolonged neurological deficits in four patients
following the epidural or accidental subarachnoid injection of large doses
of chloroprocaine have given rise to fears that this agent may be particularly neurotoxic. Studies in animals appear contradictory: chloroprocaine but not lidocaine was found to cause local toxic effects in an
isolated rabbit vagus nerve preparation, while rabbit sciatic nerves exposed to chloroprocaine for a period of six hours did not reveal any
signs of histological damage. Investigations in dogs in which chloroprocaine and bupivacaine were administered intrathecally in doses sufficient to cause total spinal anesthesia demonstrated that chloroprocaine
produced permanent paralysis in approximately 30% of the animals, whereas none of the bupivacaine-treated dogs showed evidence of permanent
neurological sequelae. Studies of a similar nature in sheep and monkeys
have failed to show any difference in neurotoxicity between chloroprocaine and other local anesthetics or control solutions. Paralysis which
was observed in rabbits following intrathecal injections of chloroprocaine
was believed to be related to sodium bisulfite, which is employed as an
antioxidant in chloroprocaine solutions. Solutions of chloroprocaine
without sodium bisulfite did not cause paralysis, whereas the sodium
bisulfite alone was associated with paralysis. More recent studies in
isolated nerves have indicated that the combination of a low pH and bisulfite may be responsible for irreversible conduction blockade rather
than the chloroprocaine itself. Nonetheless, it is obvious that special
care should be taken in performing epidural injections to avoid the accidental intrathecal injection of large amounts of local anesthetic agents.

ALLERGIC REACTIONS

Reports of allergic reactions, hypersensitivity, or anaphylactic reactions to local anesthetic agents continue to appear in the literature
periodically. Most "allergic" reactions reported by patients are actually
due to the systemic effects of epinephrine injected intravenously, though
a few may also represent minor toxic reactions to local anesthetic agents
themselves. Nonetheless, the animoester agents are capable of producing
allergic-type reactions. These agents are derivatives of paraminobenzoic
acid, which is known to be allergenic in nature, so it is logical that a
certain percentage of the population will demonstrate allergic reactions
to this class of local anesthetics. The introduction of the amino-amide
local anesthetics, which are not derivatives of paraminobenzoic acid,
markedly reduced the incidence of allergy to local anesthetic drugs.
Allergic reactions to the amino-amides are extremely rare, and while
several cases have been reported in the literature in recent years suggesting that this class of agents can on rare occasions produce an
allergic-type phenomenon, there has been only one patient reported where
the allergy to an amide local anesthetic was proven by a subsequent in-
tradermal injection of 0.2 ml of 0.5% bupivacaine, which resulted in respiratory difficulty and a decreased plasma concentration of complement
protein C_4. It should be remembered that although the amino-amide
agents appear to be relatively free from allergic reactions, solutions of
these drugs which contain methylparaben as a preservative may give rise
to allergic reactions because of the similarity of the chemical structure
of methylparaben (methy-paraminobenzoic acid).

PRESENT AND NEW APPROACHES TO REGIONAL ANESTHESIA OF THE EXTREMITIES

A.P. WINNIE

INTRODUCTION

Many anesthesiologists believe that regional anesthesia has its greatest usefulness in surgery on the extremities. A properly conducted regional technique provides operative conditions which can be matched by few other forms of anesthesia with virtually no disturbance in the function of the various organ systems. This is particularly important in patients with significant medical problems which may impose a greater threat to the patient's welfare than the condition for which he is undergoing surgery. Regional anesthesia, when properly administered, allows the surgery to be performed without significantly influencing these concomitant problems. In addition, many emergent surgical procedures on the extremities involve patients who arrive in the operating room with a full stomach. In such cases, regional anesthesia allows surgery to be performed with the patient awake, minimizing the danger of aspiration. In addition, since regional anesthesia blocks all afferent impulses arising from the site of the trauma, it abolishes the sympathetic response and any resultant tissue anoxia. Finally, all complications unique to general anesthesia are avoided when local anesthesia is used.

While many anesthesiologists agree that some form of brachial plexus block provides the best regional anesthesia for upper extremity surgery, most feel that for lower extremity surgery peripheral block anesthesia is too complicated, time consuming, and unreliable, as compared to spinal and epidural anesthesia which are simple, quick, and reliable. However, if an anesthetist is equally competent with all types of regional anesthesia, peripheral block anesthesia offers several distinct advantages; for example, postspinal headache is nonexistent, and hypotension due to preganglionic sympathetic blockade is avoided, as are the unpleasant sequelae of nausea and vomiting. Urinary retention is uncommon. Peripheral block anesthesia is particularly valuable in ambulatory surgery since it requires a much shorter postoperative recovery period and much less postoperative nursing care. With the wide choice of local anesthetic agents available today, the anesthesiologist may provide block anesthesia of 20 minutes to 12 hours duration. It even offers the surgeon varying degrees of motor blockade. Finally, in a situation where large numbers of casualties must be cared for simultaneously, peripheral nerve block permits one anesthesiologist to administer more than one anesthetic, with the monitoring carried out by less skilled members of the anesthesia care team.

If all regional anesthetics were as simple as spinals and epidurals, virtually all of the usual objections would be overcome. By its very simplicity, a single injection technique would minimize the degree of skill and experience required to perform a successful block; the time it takes to perform the block would be markedly reduced, and safety enhanced, since such complications as intravascular injection and postinjection neuropathy are known to be due to the number of injections. Because patients prefer the insertion of one rather than several needles, attempts have been made over the past decade to develop block techniques for extremity surgery at the level of the respective plexuses which innervate both the upper and the lower extremities. At this level, a single thrust of the needle identifies, not a particular nerve, but a particular fascial plane, within which the appropriate plexus lies. Injection into such an "interfascial compartment" of an appropriate volume of anesthetic allows the solution, rather than the needle, "to seek out the nerves of the plexus." In this sense, the block is similar to spinal or peridural techniques. This approach that has successfully simplified block anesthesia for surgery on both the upper and lower extremities will be discussed below.

BRACHIAL PLEXUS BLOCK

The concept of continuous perineural and perivascular space surrounding the brachial plexus from roots to terminal nerves simplifies conduction anesthesia of the upper extremity and unites the several schools of brachial block into a single school - that of perivascular anesthesia. Thus, just as with peridural techniques, the space may be entered at any level - axillary, subclavian, or interscalene - and the extent of anesthesia will depend on the volume of anesthetic and the level at which it is injected.

This concept has as its basis the fact that the brachial plexus is enveloped from the cervical vertebrae to the distal axilla by an extension of the prevertebral fascia. The prevertebral fascia splits first to invest the anterior and middle scalene muscles, forming between them an interscalene space into which the roots of the brachial (and cervical) plexus emerge from the grooved transverse processes of the cervical vertebrae. As the roots pass down through this space, they converge on the first rib to form the trunks and then divisions of the plexus, which together with the subclavian artery invaginate the scalene fascia to form a subclavian perivascular space. Passing beneath the clavicle, the divisions of the plexus split and recombine to become the cords of the plexus, and as the subclavian artery becomes the axillary, the fascia surrounding

284

the neurovascular bundle becomes the axillary sheath, which continues
into the axilla forming the axillary perivascular space.

The development of an exact technique depends not only on a knowledge of the anatomy of the brachial plexus but also on the ability to
locate this anatomy using topographic landmarks. These landmarks, however, are not bony, as previously thought, but rather muscular and
vascular. Hence, the perivascular techniques described above utilize
mainly the sense of touch. If you can palpate the interscalene groove,
the subclavian artery, and the axillary artery, you can master all of the
perivascular techniques of brachial plexus anesthesia. Which technique
is used in any case will then be determined not by the experience or
bias of the anesthetist but rather by the site of the surgery, the condition of the patient, and the level of anesthesia desired.

Axillary Perivascular Technique (Figure 1)

Our axillary perivascular technique is as follows: The patient is in
the supine position with the arm abducted 90° and the forearm flexed
and externally rotated so that the dorsum of the hand lies on the table
next to the patient's head. The axillary artery is palpated and followed
proximally as far as possible to the point where it disappears under the
pectoralis major. At this point, with the index finger directly over the
pulse, a 1½ inch 21 gauge needle is inserted just above the finger tip
toward the apex of the axilla such that it will form a 10-20° angle with
the artery as it is advanced. The artery is thus approached gradually
until the definite "click" caused by the penetration of the axillary sheath
is encountered. The tip of the needle now lies superiorly tangential to
the arterial wall 1 to ½ inches above the most proximal point of palpable
pulsation. If properly placed, the needle will clearly pulsate. Following aspiration, 20-40 ml (depending on patient's size, sex and age and

the level of anesthesia desired) of anesthetic is injected slowly with repeated aspiration for blood intermittently during the injection.

Subclavian Perivascular Technique (Figure 2)

Applying the perivascular concept to the supraclavicular approach
obviates the undesirable features of the classic technique, which is
modified as follows: The patient is in the dorsal recumbent position
with the head turned somewhat to the side opposite that to be injected.
He is told to reach for his knee (to lower the clavicle) and then to relax the arm and shoulder completely. He is then asked to elevate his
head slightly to bring the clavicular head of the sternocleidomastoid
muscle into prominence. Beginning at the lateral border of this muscle,
the index finger is rolled laterally across the belly of the anterior scalene muscle until the interscalene groove is palpated. The finger is
moved inferiorly along the groove until the pulse of the subclavian artery is palpated as it emerges from between the scalene muscles. With
the finger still on the artery, a 1½ inch 21 gauge needle is inserted
above this point in a direction that is directly caudad but not mesiad
but dorsad. The direction of insertion is such that the needle will be
dorsally tangential to the subclavian artery in the longest dimension of
the interscalene space, where the depth allows considerably more movement of the needle without its leaving the space. If the needle is advanced slowly the click of the needle penetrating the sheath may be
perceived, though it is less pronounced than that of the axillary sheath;
and a short distance beyond a single paresthesia to the hand confirms
the fact that the needle is definitely in the perivascular space. At this
point after the appropriate aspiration, the entire anesthetic injection is
made. Usually, at the beginning of the injection, "pressure anesthesia",
similar to that seen when anesthetic solution is injected rapidly into the

caudal canal, offers further evidence that the needle is properly placed.

The direction of needle insertion, the use of a short needle, and the use of a single injection not only tend to improve the incidence of satisfactory results, but also to minimize the possibility of pneumothorax. Since the direction of needle insertion is parallel to the borders of the scalene muscles and since these muscles insert on the first rib, the position of the rib and vessel is located more precisely with this technique than with any other, although with this technique, in the vast majority of cases, paresthesias are obtained before the rib has been contacted.

Interscalene Technique (Figure 3)

As pointed our earlier, as the roots of the brachial and cervical plexuses emerge from their grooved transverse processes, they enter the interscalene space formed by the fascia covering the anterior and middle scalene muscles. Since the majority of this space is above both the subclavian artery and the cupola of the lung, it would seem to be almost an ideal point to perform a brachial block at least from the point of view of safety.

The technique, as we have employed it, is as follows: The patient is in a position similar to that used in the subclavian perivascular technique. The interscalene groove is palpated, and the level of the sixth cervical vertebrae is determined by extending a line from the cricoid cartilege to the interscalene groove, and at this point, a 1½ inch, 22 gauge needle is inserted into the groove perpendicular to the skin in all planes. The direction of injection is thus slightly caudad and dorsad as well as mesiad. The needle is advanced until a paresthesia is elicited and/or the transverse process is encountered. Once a paresthesia has been evoked the desired volume of anesthetic is injected.

Lumbar Plexus Block

As with the roots of the brachial plexus, the roots of the lumbar plexus are sandwiched between two muscles, the quadratus lumborum muscle posteriorly and the psoas major muscle anteriorly, and hence at the level of its formation, the lumbar plexus is invested by the fasciae of these two muscles. Once formed, the three nerves to the leg derived from the lumbar plexus take widely divergent courses through the pelvis and into the leg, but of the three only the femoral nerve remains in close proximity to the psoas muscle throughout its descent. This nerve, which is the largest branch of the lumbar plexus, forms behind the psoas major muscle from the dorsal portions of the second, third, and fourth lumbar nerves, and descends to appear at the lateral margin of the psoas major muscle at approximately the junction of the middle and lower thirds of that muscle. However, as it continues on its course to the thigh, the femoral nerve remains in the gutter between the psoas major and the iliacus muscles so that, above the inguinal ligament, the nerve is bounded laterally by the fascia of the iliacus muscle, medially by the fascia of the psoas major muscle, and anteriorly by the transversalis fascia. In other words, in its pelvic descent towards the thigh the nerve is enveloped in a fascial extension of the compartment in which the lumbar plexus formed above the pelvic brim. As the nerve passes under the inguinal ligament into the thigh, the fused iliopsoas fascia continues to provide a posterior and lateral wall of this compartment, the inguinal ligament and, below it, the fascial lata continue to provide an anterior wall, and the thick iliopectineal fascia provides a continuation of the medial wall.

The inguinal paravascular technique of lumbar plexus block utilizes the fascial envelope around the femoral nerve as a conduit which carries injected anesthetic up to the level where the lumbar plexus forms and thus provides, with a single injection, anesthesia not only of the femoral nerve, but of the obturator and lateral femoral cutaneous nerves as well. The technique is carried out as follows: The patient is placed in the supine position, with the anesthesiologist standing on the side opposite the site of the anticipated surgery. Following the usual preparation of the skin, the anesthetist palpates the lateral edge of the femoral arterial pulse, and an "immobile needle", a short bevel, 22 gauge needle with a translucent hub connected to a syringe loaded with anesthetic, is inserted just lateral to the finger tip. The technique is carried out in a manner similar to that in which an axillary perivascular technique is carried out, with the needle sliding just over the finger tip in a cephalad direction. However, with the inguinal paravascular technique, a paresthesia of the femoral nerve must be obtained, not because a paresthesia is necessary to obtain anesthesia of the femoral nerve, but because a paresthesia indicates that the tip of the needle is placed within the perineural envelope. Following the production of a paresthesia, the needle is immobilized and the desired volume of local anesthetic is injected while firm digital pressure is applied just distal to the needle to prevent retrograde and promote cephalad spread of the agent. Following the completion of the injection, the needle is removed, but the digital pressure is maintained, with cephalad-caudad massage of the area. In an adult, the approximate appropriate volume of the anesthetic in cc's can be determined by dividing the height in inches by a factor of 3.

The clinical significance of this technique in terms of the safety, simplicity, and consistency of results that can be achieved should be readily apparent. Moore has emphasized that "open operations on or above the knee can not be carried out under the combination of sciatic

and femoral nerve blocks <u>unless</u> the lateral femoral cutaneous and obturator nerves are also blocked", and goes on to state that since even in
the most experienced hands, blocking of the obturator nerve is often unsatisfactory, if the patient's physical status dictates that regional anesthesia should be employed, we would be better to utilize spinal.

However, if an anesthesiologist is able to provide anesthesia for operations on the <u>lower</u> leg and foot with the combination of a sciatic and
femoral block, then he <u>can</u> provide anesthesia of the <u>entire</u> leg by the
same combination of the blocks <u>if</u> he simply modifies his technique of
femoral block by not injecting without paresthesias and by increasing the
volume of anesthetic injected. In other words, open operations on or
above the knee <u>can</u> be carried out under the combination of inguinal
paravascular lumbar plexus block and sciatic block.

Furthermore, the use of the inguinal paravascular technique of lumbar plexus block does more than just enhance the simplicity and increase
the extent of anesthesia: it obviously also reduces the possibility of adverse side effects, for in attempting to provide block anesthesia of all
four nerves by conventional techniques, as many as 10 to 15 insertions
of the needle may be required and as much as 65 to 95 cc of local anesthetic. As a result, the chance of complications is increased in three
ways: first, the possibility of postanesthetic neuropathy is enchanced,
since the incidence of this complication increases with the number of
times a needle penetrates a nerve; secondly, the possibility of intravascular injection increases as the number of injections increases; and
lastly, the possibility of overdosage and the appearance of signs of
systemic toxicity increases as the total volume of anesthetic injected increases. By reducing the number of injections required <u>and</u> the volume
injected, the inguinal paravascular technique virtually abolishes the

chances of complications, either neural or systemic.

Lumbosacral Plexus Block (Figure 4)

If the patient can be turned to the lateral position, and if spinal and/or epidural anesthesia are undesirable or contraindicated (the patient refuses spinal, is on anticoagulant, etc.), it is possible to block both the lumbar and sacral plexuses by a lumbar paravertebral approach. The technique is carried out in a manner that is almost identical to that which would be used to perform a paravertebral L_4 block, except that following a performance of a paresthesia, 40 cc of local anesthetic is injected. Since such an injection is made into the interfascial space between the quadratus lumborum and psoas major muscle, the solution dissects caudad and cephalad within this space to produce anesthesia of both the lumbar and sacral plexuses.

The technique is carried out as follows: The patient is placed in the lateral spinal position, lying on the side opposite that to be blocked. A line is drawn connecting the superior borders of both iliac crests, indicating the L_4-L_5 interspace, and a second line is drawn parallel to the spine, but passing through the posterior superior iliac spine. At the point where the intercrestal line crosses the paraspinous line, a 3½ inch, 22 gauge needle is inserted perpendicular to the skin, but with a slight mesiad direction. If the transverse process is encountered, the needle is redirected slightly more caudad and advanced until a paresthesia is produced. When a paresthesia has been elicited (about 5-6 centimeters beneath the skin surface) the needle is immobilized, and the injection is carried out. If the transverse process is encountered, the needle is walked off the inferior border of the transverse process until it passes beyond the process and a paresthesia is obtained.

AXILLARY PERIVASCULAR BRACHIAL PLEXUS BLOCK

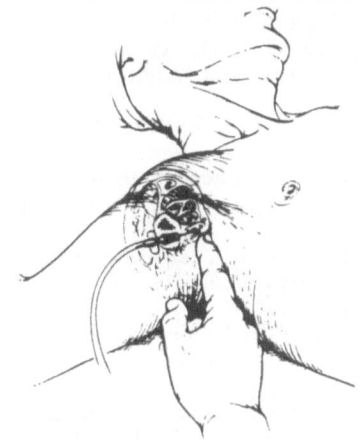

FIGURE 1: Axillary perivascular brachial plexus block as carried out by the author. A single injection is made superiorly tangential to the arterial pulse in a proximal direction to promote cephalad flow. The palpating finger collapses the vein and rolls it inferiorly during insertion of the needle to minimise the possibility of venipuncture. During the injection the finger is placed distal to the needle and digital pressure is applied to prevent retrograde flow.

SUBCLAVIAN PERIVASCULAR BRACHIAL PLEXUS BLOCK

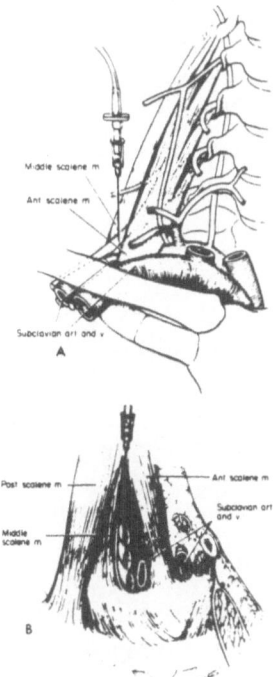

FIGURE 2: A. Frontal section showing a needle properly placed for a subclavian perivascular block. Note the directly caudad direction of the needle. B. Sagittal section showing that the caudad direction of the needle places it in the longest axis of the subclavian perivascular space. Note also that the properly placed needle lies closer to the middle scalene muscle than to the anterior scalene.

INTERSCALENE BRACHIAL PLEXUS BLOCK

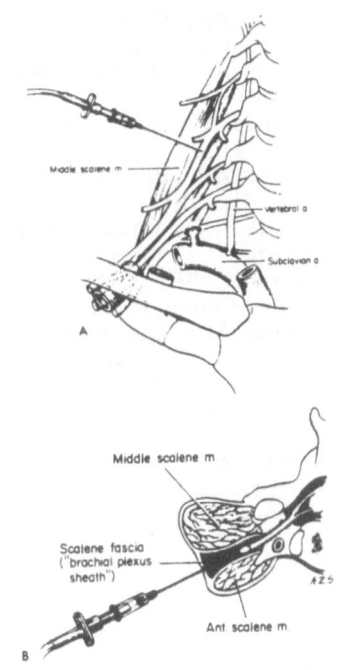

FIGURE 3: A. Frontal view showing a needle properly placed for an interscalene brachial plexus block. Note the slight caudad direction of the needle which is crucial to the prevention of a needle which has missed the roots of the plexus from entering the vertebral vessels or the epidural or subarachnoid spaces. B. Cross-sectional view showing a needle properly placed for an interscalene brachial plexus block. Note the slight dorsad direction of needle.

LUMBOSACRAL PLEXUS BLOCK

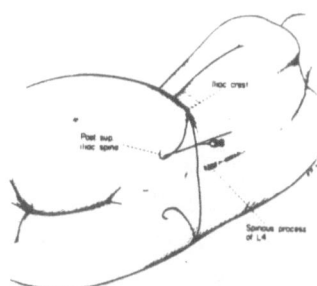

FIGURE 4: With the patient in the spinal position, a line is drawn between the two iliac crests, and a second line is drawn parallel to the spine through the posterior superior iliac spine. A 3½ inch spinal needle is inserted at the intersection of these two lines perpendicular to the skin, but with a slight mesiad direction. If the transverse process is encountered, the needle is directed slightly more caudad and advanced until a paresthesia is produced, at which point the needle is immobilized and the injection is carried out.

292

REFERENCES

1. Winnie AP, Collins VJ: The subclavian perivascular technique of brachial plexus anesthesia.   Anesthesiology 25:353-363, 1964.
2. Winnie AP: Interscalene brachial block.   Anesthesia & Analgesia 49:455-466, 1970.
3. Winnie AP: An immobile needle for nerve blocks.   Anesthesiology 31:577-578, 1969.
4. Winnie AP, Radonjic R, Akkineni SR, Durrani Z: Factors influencing distribution of local anesthetic injected into the brachial plexus sheath.   Anesthesia & Analgesia 58:225-234, 1979.
5. Winnie AP: Plexus Anesthesia I: The Perivascular Technique of Brachial Plexus Block.   W.B. Saunders Company, Philadelphia and Schultz Medical Information ApS, Copenhagen, 1983.
6. Winnie AP, Ramamurthy S, Durrani Z: The inguinal paravascular technic of lumbar plexus anesthesia.   Anesthesia & Analgesia 52:989-996, 1973.
7. Winnie AP, Ramamurthy S, Durrani Z, Radonjic R: Plexus blocks for lower extremity surgery.   Anesthesiology Review 1:11-16, 1974.
8. Winnie AP: Regional Anesthesia for Surgery on the Extremities.   Chapter 6 in Anesthesia for Orthopaedic Surgery.   Edited by Zauder HL, Philadephia, F.A. Davis Company, 1980, pp. 89-117.